IN PRAISE OF
FROM UNBECOMING A NURSE TO OVERCOMING ADDICTION

"Who heals the healers? In Paula Davies Scimeca's first book, Unbecoming a Nurse, we learned that even the most conscientious nurses can succumb to the pressures - and temptations - of a demanding, exacting profession. In this, Scimeca's second book, we learn how they fight back and conquer their addictions.

"The personal narratives of nurses in recovery from addiction are straightforward, explicit, and startlingly frank. Some are graceful; some are blunt, but all are eye-openers. Scimeca's decision to allow the nurses to tell their stories, in their own words, and from their unique perspective was a significant one. Her extensive knowledge of, and respect for, the nursing profession is the driving force behind her book. She not only empowered those telling the stories, but lent credence to their accounts. By withholding editorial comments, Scimeca permits the voices to ring true and uncontrived, thus loudly proclaiming that recovery is not only possible, but probable. This book brings long overdue support to vulnerable nurses and their families."

Jennie L. Brown, author *Blue Moon Rising: Kentucky Women in Transition*

"What a beautiful and powerful book that Scimeca has weaved together! In our lives as recovering people and our work as recovery advocates, we know firsthand the stigma and discrimination faced by women and men who live in recovery. The ravages of stigma breed in silence, behind closed doors and become real barriers for those needing help to stop addiction in its tracks. What Scimeca has done is shine a light in those dark places and give voice to the real-life struggles and successes of nurses who commit themselves to recovery. These stories demonstrate what we know: that people with alcohol and drug addiction can be freed through recovery and live well. The more we publicize this fact, the more individuals and families who suffer from addiction can find their way to recovery."

Deb Dettor, Coordinator, Maine Alliance for Addiction Recovery

"A book for nurses that creates enlightenment for all, *From Unbecoming A Nurse To Overcoming Addiction* will save many from a disease that all believe will never affect them. It should be required reading for every healthcare professional to ensure preconceptions are replaced with understanding and comprehension of a disease that has no preference for social or professional standing. Hopefully this book will save some nurses from the pain of walking in the shoes of an addict."

Larry Golbom, RPh, MBA, host of The Prescription Addiction Radio Show – Breaking The Silence

"This book profiles courage and is a resource for nurses who suffer from alcohol and/or substance abuse, or have colleagues suffering with an addictive disease. It is enlightening, poignant and in moments humorous. This book helps raise awareness and informs a better understanding of the disease process of addiction."

Deborah Egel, RN, CARN, Esq.

"This book should be required reading for all nurse training programs, state boards of nursing, alternative to discipline program staff and employers. The stigma associated with chemical dependence prevents those struggling with the disease from seeking and/or accepting help. Stigma arises from the lack of knowledge, and training programs provide little, if any, education regarding the disease of addiction. Paula has provided the nursing profession with practical information that is immediately useful. She has also shown us the human side of those nurses trapped in the downward spiral that is addiction. If we hope to reverse the alarming rise in the numbers of people becoming dependent on prescription medications, especially in children whose age of first use is eleven to twelve years of age, we must educate our society regarding the disease of chemical dependence. Since nurses are the front line health care providers, it makes sense to begin this education in the nursing profession. After all, if nurses don't understand this disease or recognize it in their colleagues, how can we expect the rest of society to do any better?"

Jack Stem, CEO & Founder of Peer Advocacy For Impaired Nurses, LLC

"This book offers a view into the hearts and minds of those whose lives have been influenced by addiction. These stories help us all understand how we can change, grow, and successfully live in recovery. Thank you for giving voice to their experiences."
Kate Driscoll Malliarakis, RN, CNP, MAC, Pres., KAM Associates

"Paula Scimeca has managed with this book to address this most serious problem of nurses and addiction through the words of the addicts themselves. This provides us with a concentrated source of understanding and insight that would take perhaps months or years to gather otherwise. It is enlightening and useful to both the clinician helping the addicted nurse and hopefully, the addict, who will learn that he or she does not struggle alone."
E'Louise Ondash, RN/Author

IN PRAISE OF
UNBECOMING A NURSE

"I am a nurse attorney who has for the past twenty years represented nurses and other healthcare professionals in licensure disciplinary cases. In my opinion, Paula's book, *Unbecoming A Nurse*, serves as a valuable tool for all nurses and nursing students... I have personally read the book several times and can say that with each read, I gain some additional insight into the issues surrounding addiction. I highly recommend this book to all nurses."
Karen J. Halpern, RN, BSN, MSN, JD

"My son was a Registered Nurse. He was a wonderful, caring and compassionate young man. He loved taking care of people, especially the elderly... Sadly, he was also a drug addict. Scimeca's book *Unbecoming A Nurse* is a must read for anyone connected to the nursing profession no matter how closely or remotely."
Sheryl Letzgus McGinnis, author, *I Am Your Disease: The Many Faces of Addiction*

"I became interested in the subject matter of *Unbecoming A Nurse* as a result of my position on the New York State Professional Assistance Committee (PAP)... I truly believe that *Unbecoming A Nurse* should have a place in the nursing curriculum and is a must read for anyone thinking about becoming a nurse or anyone who lives with or loves a nurse."
John W. Mullen

From
UNBECOMING
a NURSE to
OVERCOMING
ADDICTION

Candid Self-Portraits of

Nurses in Recovery

Paula Davies Scimeca, RN, MS

Published by Sea Meca, Inc.
P.O. Box 090455
Staten Island, New York 10309-0455
www.unbecominganurse.org
Printed in the United States of America

Library of Congress Control Number: 2010901735

ISBN 978-0-9821904-1-8

Dedication

This book is dedicated to Rachel B. and Priscilla I., whom I have never met, but who, in my estimation, displayed the ultimate refinement of character described in the literature of Alcoholics Anonymous. May they both rest in peace as surely as they continue to inspire those they have left behind.

Acknowledgments

My heartfelt gratitude to all the nurses who made this book vividly come to life by graciously and candidly giving the priceless gift of themselves. It is my firmest conviction that your individual contribution of experience with addiction and in recovery, combined with your collective strength, hope and wisdom, will offer comfort, support, guidance and inspiration to nurses ensnared in their own nightmarers. Hopefully, by so courageously and generously illuminating the path you took, not only the downward spiral but the road to recovery, others may avoid the anguish you suffered, either totally or in part. God bless each and every one of you!

A warm note of thanks to Bill B. for sharing Rachel's story in such a compelling manner as well as Ken I. for sharing so poignantly Priscilla's journey with us.

To Thomas, for continuing to buoy me up, not just financially but physically and emotionally throughout this project. Thank you for all you have endured without complaint and for greeting me each and every day with ongoing smiles. As always, you are a far better husband than I am a wife.

To Tara, John, Melissa, Michelle, Kathy and Dot for lending ongoing assistance, support and the brightest of smiles.

The list of colleagues, friends and family who supported me in this endeavor is incredibly long, but I must send a special note of thanks to those in the International Nurses Society on Addictions and the International Womens' Writing Guild for all the kind words of encouragement throughout this lengthy and at times arduous project.

My list would be incomplete without crediting Divine Destiny for, once again, giving me a persistent vision of this book. Certainly any ability or willingness to begin, let alone complete this volume, never emanated solely from me.

Table of Contents

Although the world is full of suffering,

It is also full of the overcoming of it.

Helen Keller

Introduction

Tragically, there is a mounting toll exacted from society by addiction each and every day, not just in United States but around the globe. Nowhere does this issue strike a more critical blow than upon the very heart and soul of the nursing profession. While the specific dimensions of its impact remain unquantifiable, it is indeed a profound and persistent phenomenon which can harm not just the nurses themselves, but their families, friends, colleagues, employers and patients.

Desperately trying to hide, maintain, relieve or recover from their addiction, several thousand nurses annually face their most formidable challenge: a hidden trap they never dreamed they would meet, let alone endure. Blindsided and spellbound in the grip of chemical dependency and process addictions such as gambling, eating disorders and codependency, those afflicted with addiction undergo the ultimate shift from the pursuit of happiness each were born with, to an unquenchable quest for mood-altering substances and behaviors. While some nurses follow this craving until stripped of their liberty and others spiral down to surrender their privilege to practice nursing, more tragic still are those swindled of their very lives.

Nevertheless, this is a book of hope. It chronicles the descent of twenty-nine nurses into a nightmarish quagmire beyond compare. Their stories attest to the fact that addiction has no respect for any personal or professional distinctions. Hailing from twenty states, various social backgrounds and a wide array of nursing specialties, each account portrays an utter inability to extricate oneself from addiction in spite of exquisite suffering and tremendous loss.

While many of the nurses depict continuous recoveries lasting decades, others point a laser beam at the factors which preceded a relapse. Offering their hindsight, they have detailed the finer points of recovery which were either missed or disregarded in prior attempts and they go on to expound upon specific actions they now take to avoid any future ambush.

The book concludes with two inspirational testimonies shared by the husbands of Rachel and Priscilla who poignantly describe their wives' uninterrupted recoveries of nineteen and thirty-five years, respectively. Though Rachel and Priscilla's journeys on earth have been cut short by cancer, their recoveries have proven to be long-lasting and permanent; examples of remissions which endured, intact, and remained sufficiently resilient to withstand not only the test of time but terminal illness.

These twenty-nine compelling profiles of nurses in recovery offer an enormous wealth of priceless life experience and lessons-learned; a treasure trove of wisdom ordinarily overshadowed by the more sensational media headlines regarding nurse drug diversion and prescription forgery. Since most nurses tend to "guard their anonymity with their life," as one nurse put it, the blossoms of recovery sprouting quietly to life all around us usually remain a miracle few are privy to; yet many would give anything to latch hold of.

In an age when so many wonders are taken for granted and good news is in very short supply, these candid reflections inspire all who may be in search of their own miracle. Nurse faculty, employers, substance abuse professionals and policymakers can also benefit from these candid illustrations which clearly demonstrate the seemingly subtle, yet often crucial, nuances which either help or hinder a nurse's road to uninterrupted and continuous recovery.

Truly, my ultimate privilege as a nurse has been to serve as a conduit for these stories from nurses in recovery who very graciously entrusted me with their innermost thoughts, gut-wrenching feelings, harrowing escapades and miraculous journeys, expressly for this publication. In my estimation, each one of them exposed the barest essence of themselves, heart and soul, throughout the following pages.

While many variables exist regarding their innate beliefs and actual experiences, a common thread is intricately woven throughout each narrative. Clearly, crisply, cleanly, as a scalpel cutting strategically through their darkest moments and greatest accomplishments, is the unmistakably heartfelt intent of each contributor to lend their experience, strength and hope of recovery in order that others may reap some benefit.

Somewhere in every nurse lies the realization that within each of us is the very greatest gift we can ever bestow on another human being. While that notion is mirrored throughout this book, each story also reflects the ultimate recognition that, along with the ability to minister to others both personally and professionally, come the unavoidable responsibility to self-nurture, preserve and protect that precious, priceless inner-self.

Although the tragic consequences of addiction are real and at times lethal, scattered throughout these pages are some ironic, if not humorous, anecdotal comments from nurses describing their journey. For any who may have experienced the loss of their own beloved nurse due to addiction or who may have suffered at the hands of an impaired caregiver, I offer the following quote from the book, "Alcoholics Anonymous," to explain what may appear, at first blush, to be a flippant or impertinent demeanor.

3

"When we see a man sinking into the mire that is alcoholism, we give first aid and place what we have at his disposal. For his sake, we recount and almost relive the horrors of our past. But for those of us who have tried to shoulder the entire burden and trouble of others find we are soon overcome by them.

So we think cheerfulness and laughter make for usefulness. Outsiders are sometimes shocked when we burst into merriment over a seemingly tragic experience out of the past. But why shouldn't we laugh? We have recovered, and have been given the power to help others." Alcoholics Anonymous, Fourth Edition, page 132.

In closing, I must admit that as a child who once had Olympic aspirations, I held in the very highest regard a strikingly beautiful woman who later became my coach and mentor. In awestruck wonder of her winning not just one, but two gold medals in Rome in 1960, I emulated her and worked very hard to become the best I could be at our chosen sport.

Having applied similar stellar efforts to many other endeavors over the years personally, academically and professionally, I currently find myself well past the midpoint of my life. Becoming a nurse stands out as having been the pivotal catalyst which has afforded me a rewarding life as well as a fulfilling career that, upon reflection, shows many a mistake but only one true regret.

Today, with a much keener vision of what truly constitutes courage and qualities worth emulating, profiling and praising, my very highest admiration and respect is solely reserved for the nurses whose stories of recovery grace these pages and the thousands of other nurses who accompany them on their journey, one day at a time.

Someone Must Have Prayed For Me

Growing up, I thought "partying" was what you were supposed to do. My father worked all week, my mother stayed home and when the weekend came around they were off to the clubs. There wasn't much emphasis put on school; only that it was where we went when available to "get out of our mother's hair."

My family moved a lot. Between my father's trouble with the law and his general discontent with life on life's terms, we moved between two and four times a year.

As a child, I did not realize I was living in a very dysfunctional home; it was my norm. A lot of verbal and emotional abuse went on in our home which, coupled with the constant moving, laid the ground-work for a very insecure teenager with very low self-worth. I began to experiment with drugs as a preteen.

Needless to say, as a teen I wanted out, and so I left home as a runaway at fourteen. I lived with a nineteen year-old boyfriend for six or so months, at which time I became introduced to all sorts of drugs and alcohol. I was well on my way to becoming a full-fledged addict.

When I was fifteen, my boyfriend and I split up and I lived on my own in a trailer for awhile. Then I moved to an abandoned farm house. I worked at a restaurant for a time before being picked up by a local sheriff for being a runaway.

My parents came to retrieve me, only to take me home and, after three days, loaded me up and dropped me off at the bus station after buying me a one-way bus ticket back to the town my abandoned farm house was in.

Now I was really on a downhill slide. I returned to the abandoned farm house where my addiction became my best friend and my endless pursuit. It was during this next year that I became introduced to IV methamphetamine, crank as we called it. This started an addiction that spanned over thirteen years.

As an IV drug addict, I made many wrong choices, many which landed me in trouble with the law. I have spent my share of time in jail, only to be released and go back on the addiction train.

Being a drug addict was not what I wanted to be, but I was in a trap in which I could not find a way out. I wanted out and, at times, remember wishing I would go to jail because it was the only way I could stop the endless pursuit of obtaining and self-administering drugs.

Something inside me (today I know it was God) was telling me if I did not stop I was going to die. It was so profound that I knew I had to find a way out of this addiction trap, or I was indeed going to die. Even so, I could not stop.

Today I know somewhere, at sometime, someone must have prayed for me. Was it the youth minister who recruited child-ren for youth group from one of the apartments where I had lived as a child? It is to this man that I credit my relationship with God. Or was it one of the women who prayed with me on a street corner where I hung out as a runaway teen in California? Maybe they both had pleaded to God for me.

So, here I am in this death trap, knowing in my core that I am going to die if I don't get out; yet I cannot find a way out. I ask God to PLEASE make a way out of this trap for me. I confess to Him that I know I am going to die, but that I do not want to die; that I want to live and contribute to society.

Not long after that, on one of my "drug runs," I am arrested again. Only this time is different; I am placed in a drug rehab. I had never even heard of drug rehabs or AA, NA, 12 steps or anything like that before. I did not even know anybody who didn't use drugs.

"Wow, this is it," I thought, "God's made a way out for me!" I latched onto recovery like a drowning victim to a life pre-server. I said to myself, "I am going to give this everything I have and if it doesn't work, I will just die."

Amazingly enough, it works! Praise God is all I can say. Something magical happens when you turn it all over to God and work those 12 steps to the best of your ability.

I came into recovery with an 8th grade education and a head full of street survival knowledge, which is useless in the responsible, real world. I spent the first year in a drug rehab, going from inpatient to a halfway house and then to a sober living community. I was a long-term addict and needed long-term rehab.

In the second year of my recovery, I got my GED and from there applied to and got accepted into LPN/LVN school. Life had been waiting on me.

The Board of Nursing in my state made me "jump through a lot of hoops" because of my history of arrest to earn the privilege of being a nurse. But this has turned out to be a God deal.

First of all, in my early days working as an LPN, I had to work a program with the nursing board's Peer Assistance Program.

7

This program helped me remain steady in my recovery and focus on my calling to be a nurse. I am a huge Peer Assistance fan.

My nursing career has been very rewarding and challenging. Today, I am an RN with a Masters degree in Nursing Education and teach nursing to practical nursing students.

I have a wonderful husband and three great children. I have been clean and sober for over sixteen years now and not a day goes by that I don't reflect on how grateful I am to be alive and living an abundant life.

I am very active in things pertaining to my recovery. My life depends on it. I am also a committee member with our Board of Nursing's Peer Assistance Committee.

The disease of addiction is still alive and it still wants to kill me; but as long as I don't use, I don't have to worry about it. For me, recovery is all about giving myself to God and surrendering to the fact that I am powerless over anything mind altering. Denial or trying to justify or rationalize the use of mind altering substances is a deadly trap for me.

Working the 12 steps of recovery is a prescription for life to me. I will always be "in recovery." My disease is never cured, only in remission. So I live my life one day at a time, sometimes one minute at a time; whatever pace it takes to keep my focus on the necessity of staying clean and sober. Recovery works, if you work it.

From Twisted Path To The Triumph Of Recovery

I am a nurse who has always lived on the edge. I'm a retired Colonel in the Army Nurse Corps who served on active duty in the U.S. Army reserves over a thirty-four year span. My last assignment on active duty was the chief nurse in Dessert Storm/Gulf War at King Khalid Military City, which was located on the Iraq /Kuwait border.

Looking back, I came from an environment where there was always drinking and gambling. The town I grew up in was very small, about a mile square. Believe it or not, it had as many churches as it had barrooms and bookie joints.

My mother was an alcoholic and I had no father. At seven-and-a-half, I delivered my sister. I was the little girl going about, taking my mother out of the barrooms by the time I was eight. I was also the kid who had to say my father died, when he really didn't die, to protect my sister.

I loved my mother because she was my only parent and I hated her because she was an alcoholic. I always said I would never be like my mother. Although I didn't start drinking heavily until I was about thirty-two years of age, I went on to become like her. I finally ended my drinking at age forty-two.

Growing up in poverty, in a cold-water flat, I never knew what it was like to have a shower in the home. The local Boy's Club had a girl's night where we showered, so I made it work. I was always able to make it work.

Although I did not drink or get drunk every day, I started drinking at fourteen. People would always try to find out where I was. They knew that if there was a party, it would be wherever I was. That gave me an identity and I loved it.

9

I was also introduced to gambling at a very young age, which somehow always made me feel I was special, and older, which I liked. Gambling also gave me excitement, so when I was bored, I always went gambling. Of course, I did not gamble my way through life early, but I certainly dabbled in it, on and off. Looking back now, I can see that I couldn't deal with boredom or the feeling of emptiness, so I compensated by creating some sort of excitement. That excitement came when I gambled.

While I always thought I could control the alcohol and control the gambling, I was always afraid to use drugs. I don't actually know why, but because I had that fear, I never even smoked a joint.

At fifteen, I was hired as a domestic for a wealthy family. I went on to work in many other places, even on tuna derbies. Alcohol really infiltrated everything I did.

Deciding to become a nurse, I chose a career in the military, where there was also a lot of drinking. I was a combat nurse who always worked in ICU or emergency rooms. On the civilian side of the house, I worked in the newborn intensive care units. Just about everything I did in nursing was dealing with some type of emergency situation, like the codes and the fast pace that goes along with that environment.

I thrived on all that "Let's move it, let's move it, let's go!" type of nursing. I was really addicted to the adrenalin rush that those situations created, even though I really didn't know that for a long time.

Strictly a party girl who was drinking in barrooms, I was able to carry the identity I had growing up along with me into the military. Even though I wasn't one to drink at home, I was secretive about how much I drank. If I went to anything professionally, I would only have a few drinks and then I would leave to really have some fun.

Eventually, alcoholism, like any addiction, takes away that part of you that has the ability to make a decision of either "Yeah" or Nay." I can remember so clearly when that happened to me, because I said to myself, "My God. Your choices are getting worse and worse."

Like the choice of what to drink if I got up at three in the morning, dying of thirst after being out drinking the evening before. I would have to decide whether I was going to have a glass of juice or a beer. On occasions when I decided to take a beer instead of the juice, I wouldn't go to work in the morning. So, my alcoholism took me to a point where it affected my attendance and my work. Like any addiction, it was progressive.

When I got in trouble, I went on sabbaticals from work and left the military. I ended up in a halfway house in 1978, financially and spiritually broken. I felt I had lost my military career. I had lost my position as a head nurse in a neonatal intensive care unit just prior to that and had taken time out because I was getting the shakes and all that goes along with alcoholism.

That's when I realized that I had to choose whether I wanted to be a nurse or a bum. I decided that I wanted to be a nurse and get back into the military. At that point, I found myself looking in the bin of donations at the halfway house for a pair of white nursing shoes to get back on duty. I got on my knees like we are told to do and asked God to give me the strength, the courage and hope, to get my life back together.

Over time, I got everything I prayed for. I got an apartment, a car and a great job. I also got a letter from the Pentagon saying that they had reviewed my records and had made the determination that I was a good, capable nurse who would be accepted back into the Army Nurse Corps.

Actually, I got that letter at a time when I had gone back out for a few months. I returned to drinking because I did not realize that alcoholism is a progressive, chronic disease. When I got that letter from the military accepting me back, I saw it as a clear message for me to get my act together. So I entered recovery on September 21st of 1978, when I made the decision and commitment to myself that I was going to give this program an opportunity to work in me and help me. Was it hard? You bet your life it was hard!

When people saw me after I sobered up, they would often say, "God, you look wonderful." I would tell them, "Well, I don't drink anymore." Since I had hidden my alcoholism so well, they would usually say, "You never drank much." Like many other nurses, I hid my drinking very well.

Because I surrendered to win, I remain in recovery from drinking to this day. I wanted to win and to find out who I was, so I sobered up and did just that. My life got better. I was someone who had gotten every possible opportunity that one could ever have in life to better themselves and I took full advantage of each opportunity that came my way. My wildest dreams came true. Everything that I could ever want or imagine happened.

Then in 2000, at the age of sixty-three, I was no longer that Colonel in the Army Nurse Corps. I was no longer that outstanding neonatal case manager that I had become. I was no longer taking care of those really sick babies, transitioning

12

them to home, many of them still on life support. Everything was changing. On top of all that, I had gotten ovarian cancer.

Now, I certainly didn't say at the time, "OK, God, save me and I am going to go gamble all my money away." On the contrary, after my cancer treatment was successful, I became a very grateful, humble person who realized the huge impact that ovarian cancer has on women. Yet, I was never prepared for the feeling that I was losing my identity at age sixty-three.

Although I had no conscious awareness of it, the only identity I had left was gambling. I used to love to play the horses when I was younger because that was a day at the races to me. Back then, there were no ATM machines and you couldn't just cash a check. If you went with thirty dollars and lost your money, you either borrowed from a friend or you went home. Gambling was never as potentially destructive back then as it has become today.

So, when I walked into the casino in 2000, there was now the ability to get instant money. I became addicted very quickly and went through a lot of money in a very short period of time. The woman who had been the struggling young girl, who grew up in poverty, delivered her sister, worked as a domestic to get into nursing and had worked her whole life to get ahead, was now going through all her money, her 401k and investment funds, like a nut, like a screwball. Emptying out my Paine Weber fund, I actually went through roughly three hundred thousand dollars.

If someone had told me that I would display this type of behavior, I would say, "Are you crazy? I have too much respect for myself." I didn't understand the addictive component of gambling within a person nor did I understand what was within me. Even though I did not go back to drinking, I was clinging to character defects in myself that I never dealt with. I was still that little girl with a lot of fear, insecurity, emptiness and loneliness.

I never realized that my old behaviors were the strings from my childhood that I used to fill a void which ultimately became ropes I clung to. So, when I had nothing else to do, I would gamble. Now, why wouldn't I go knit a sweater like some people? Because when others were knitting argyle socks in nursing school, I was the one who never got beyond the heel.

Although I knew on a conscious level that gambling wasn't good for me, subconsciously I honestly felt I could control gambling again. So, at some point, I believed I could go into the casino with a certain number of dollars. I thought I would be able to leave if I lost or leave when I won. Eventually, I couldn't do that at all.

It wasn't until this last time that I went out that I realized I had a problem deep within my soul. I'm now going to a therapist who has helped me really go back into my childhood to understand why I did what I did. It took me awhile to truly see that I was addicted to excitement. I am addicted to the adrenalin rush without ever having taken drugs. I was a drinker, and then I was a gambler. That seemed to give me all I needed without ever taking drugs.

Since I haven't had a drink in thirty-one years, people have said to me, "Well, if you stopped drinking thirty-one years ago, why can't you just stop gambling?" Part of the reason is that I didn't fully accept that I have an addictive problem with gambling. I thought I was in control. It was my money. I wasn't stealing from anyone. I thought I was different.

14

I had what is really an attitude of entitlement. I felt I had an entitlement to do what I want. I realize now that although I do have an entitlement, I do not have an entitlement to destroy myself.

Compulsive gambling is a very subtle disease. Gambling seems to offer a home away from home, where you can go, sit at a machine and not be bothered by anyone. It does all that without you ever knowing that the gambling is taking you over mentally and also going to stop you from living. I had to learn for myself that when I am gambling, I no longer have a life.

When my drinking got to the point that I didn't have any control over liquor, it affected my mind, my gait and my behavior. If I took a drink, I'd smell of alcohol. On the other hand, gambling can be hidden better because my gait is not affected. Unless I smell of cigarette smoke from the casino, there is no detectable smell with gambling and the only thing I had to do to cover that up after spending time at the casino was to keep a change of clothes in the car.

Drinking is looked at very differently than gambling. How many times do you hear nurses say they are going to a casino to have dinner, catch a show and do a little gambling? Yet, one out of ten will eventually go on to gamble alone, without wanting to go to dinner or see the show. That's the person who wants to play the game and is hooked on the excitement of gambling. That is the individual who thinks they can get back on top.

Compulsive gamblers come to the point where they could win fifty thousand dollars one night and walk out later that same night losing sixty thousand. That is the person like me, who is

15

not gambling to win but is gambling to experience the excitement it gives them.

Today, I am very involved in AA and GA. I'm not embarrassed to tell anyone I drank too much and I eventually gambled too much. I accept the fact that I had to do what I had to do to be where I am today. From being in a halfway house in 1978 taking white shoes out of a bin, I went on to become a full colonel who addressed all the big brass in the Pentagon in 1991, representing all women who were in combat in the Gulf War. I was there to say that there is a place in combat for selected women with selected experience, such as nurses and those on medical teams.

We nurses are all very good people who sacrifice our lives in so very many ways for others, but don't know how to take care of ourselves. Many nurses have addictions, whether it is alcohol, or drugs, or gambling, or overeating. I realize that better than most nurses. Hopefully, my story will help someone else because there are other nurses out there with stories just like mine.

If I look at everything that has happened in my life, it is worth every penny to be able to be where I am today at seventy-three. I have a mission today that excites me, which is to spearhead recognition of women veterans in my state. I remain a consultant in the newborn intensive care unit and make good money. I have a beautiful home and a wonderful family. Today, I have my dignity.

Living life on life's terms more than at any other time in my life, I am learning how to just be quiet in my own soul. I understand more than ever before that it is the power of God which lifts me up. My mind is clear today to see the miracles and to see those less fortunate than me. I truly hope that I am there to help them.

So I say to God, "Keep me going and I will share everything I have." Like that little energizer bunny, as long as God keeps winding me up, I will keep sharing everything I have.

Twenty-Two Years Beyond My Wildest Dreams

Fortunately for me, I did not come into nursing with chemical dependency being a hidden trap for me. I came into the nursing community with my chemical dependency in remission.

I come from a working class Jewish family with all of the cultural denial that, in my experience, many Jewish families have. When we would talk about drinking, or whatever, it was always happening to those "other people." But the reality was that there was a multi-generational history of addictive disorders, at least on my father's side of the family.

I grew up as a very bright and curious, but angry adolescent, who in many senses felt disconnected. I learned how to drink where you're supposed to get religious training, which was in the synagogue. At age twelve or thirteen, I remember coming home from one of the bar or bas mitzvahs that my friends were having, absolutely ossified, and loving it.

After hitting the wine and schnapps at the Oneg Shabbatt, which is the Welcoming the Sabbath, I can literally remember walking over a cement bridge that was swaying back and forth on my way home, thinking that I truly had found God. It certainly was not the God that I was being taught about in synagogue, but the alcohol that had been served.

The penetration of the disease in the family, at least in retrospect, is very clear to me. One of my clearest remembrances of my Mom early-on was at my fifth birthday party. The kids were all driving her crazy in the house, so she stepped into the powder-room to chug-a-lug half a bottle of butalbital elixir. I also remember all of my aunts sharing their drugs, their benzodiazepines, sedative-hypnotics, and psychostimulants at the Passover table.

By the time I hit high school, I was pretty much a daily drinker and drug-user who basically drank and drugged my way through high school. For me, my booze bone was connected to my drug bone, which was connected to my nicotine bone.

The good and the bad news was that I was a very academically talented student. Because I did well in standardized testing, I would get suspended in the morning and then readmitted in the afternoon, without having to go home to tell my parents. I ended up dropping out of high school and getting a GED because school was interfering with my drinking and drugging.

I had a very rapid progression of my disease with multiple overdoses, treatment experiences and psychiatrists. All of the classical approaches of the 1960s and early 1970s were used regarding how to control adolescents without anyone recognizing that the primary issue that needed to be addressed was the disease of chemical dependency. It was always about getting at some other root cause without addressing the predominant symptom, which was how to control my drinking and drugging.

With my disease in quasi-remission, I ended up finally going to college. I was predominantly using prescription drugs at that point. I went into an honors' program in psycho-pharmacology and, low and behold, wound up in a laboratory doing addiction research. My research was looking at the activation and maintenance of the opioid addiction cycle, its effect on the brain and its destruction of the brain's reward track. So here I was, an honor student on a grant, with a two-and-a-half gram per day morphine habit; the biggest rat in the lab, doing addiction research.

After a number of failed treatment attempts, since my preparation was in pre-pharmacy, I began working in retail pharmacy. Much like most of the fog I lived in, I don't know how I got there, but I ended up working for a very crooked pharmacist. So I became a consultant to some folks in what I'll call "medicinal chemistry."

At the time, the Drug Enforcement Agency had begun to track all the major industrial pharmaceutical precursors for the manufacture of amphetamine-based drugs. I ended up essentially as the lab rat/consultant to this group of shady businessmen who wanted to manufacture massive quantities of these precursors. These were the products that the DEA thought were better handled by the pharmaceutical industry.

I came to find out that I was under surveillance by the DEA. I freaked out and had a death-defying overdose, ended up in the ICU and then went underground. The DEA wanted to talk with me and when I went to speak with them, I found that they had surveillance pictures of me.

The DEA basically gave me two choices: to be an unindicted co-conspirator who would testify before a grand jury; or be an indicted co-conspirator who would face five to fifteen years in prison for each count of conspiracy to manufacture and distribute controlled substances. I did not particularly like either of these choices.

At the time, I was actually living in my aunt's basement, hiding out in an absolute stupor. I was in a state of total paranoia, using anything that I could get my hands on, when I had this epiphany that this bad Jewish boy should get the hell out of the country and go to Israel to dodge the DEA.

I have no idea where this idea came from, but I went down to apply for a passport in the same federal building where I had just met with the DEA. How grandiose I was, thinking that the DEA had me, this pipsqueak that I was, under constant surveillance and knew everything I was doing, like getting a passport.

Two weeks later, I went back to that same federal building to pick up my passport, again knowing, in my grandiosity, that the DEA was going to be there to take me away in handcuffs. The reality was that I got my passport and very shortly afterwards got on a plane to Athens and then Tel Aviv.

I was scared enough in Israel to keep my addictive tendencies reasonably under control, getting whatever stuff I could get without major risk while over there. I had a couple of really intrepid drunks and remember one night drinking palm liquor and barfing my guts up under a tree near the volunteer barracks on the kibbutz. This was truly one of the worst drunks of my life.

In the meantime, I was sending fervent letters from Israel to the woman I had been engaged to back home who had broken up with me. I was telling her that I loved her, that I was a good boy and I'd learned my lesson.

After about ten or eleven months in the kibbutz, I had learned that the case with the DEA had fallen through and they were no longer pursuing it. So, after a year in the kibbutz, I left to come back to the U.S.

The thing that really shook my tree and got me serious about getting sober and getting appropriate treatment was that I was back home only one day when the person I had consulted for found me at my parents' house.

When I got summoned to meet the people who had solicited my services in a Howard Johnson's not far from my parents' place, they were trying to twist my arm. It is unbelievable, and had to be Providence, because I don't have the kind of courage to say, "No." So it wasn't me who said the words, "No. I can't do this and please don't ever contact me again." I was not built strongly enough to do that, but I walked out of there and that was the last I ever heard from them.

After treatment, I wanted to do what every good recovering addict and alcoholic does: I wanted to become a treatment professional and give back to the community. I had all of the pink cloud enthusiasm that happens in early recovery. I became a group and family therapist, a certified addiction counselor, and part of the clinical staff providing treatment services to addicts.

Then, a number of years later, like every other area of my life that's permeated by the restlessness of being an alcoholic, it was time to do something new and different. That's when I ended up going back to school and becoming a Physician's Assistant.

After I started working as a PA, I stopped going to meetings. I had a legitimate pain issue, multilevel cervical disc disease, and wasn't sleeping. I was overwhelmed with it all, so I went to my doctor to get something to help me sleep. I thought with a couple of nights' sleep that I'd be fine. The doctor wrote a prescription for six half-milligram tablets of Ativan for me and I was off to the races.

Within eighteen months, it was as if I had never breathed a sober breath in my entire life. Being the manipulative drug addict that I was, I had access to a lot of pharmaceutical reps so I was able to get them to open their trunks and give me whatever I wanted. I knew exactly what I was doing.

Finally, it got to a point when my twins were about sixteen months old that I could no longer work or I just couldn't face the work. So I was discharged from my job and went out on disability. I deluded myself that it was depression and went to see a shrink, which was great. I was a fisherman and the shrink was a fisherman. We would talk and he would write me prescriptions for one-milligram Xanax tablets in quantities of one hundred twenty pills at a time with five refills.

I would go back to see the shrink two weeks later and at the end of the session he would ask if I was OK with scripts. Was I supposed to say "Yes?" So he would write me more prescriptions. The responsibility of what I was doing was entirely mine; but he was giving me the choice to continue doing what I was doing.

Eventually, I got to a place where I was so completely useless that I would lie on the couch having crying jags about what a horrible husband and father I was; but I couldn't peel myself off the couch to walk up the steps to help with the children.

The emotional pain got to the point where no amount of drugs did anything. I took literally handfuls and handfuls of drugs and washed them down with one hundred proof vodka and it did nothing. I would fall into a stupor, drool on myself, and wake up with this screaming between my ears. The emotional agony of the committee meeting inside my head, telling me what a useless, festering bedsore I was on the butt of society was awful.

This went on into the fall of 1987 until the evening of October 20th. I ended up actually sitting at my kitchen table that night with a loaded 357 in my mouth, cocked, ready to pull the trigger. I just couldn't take another minute of living the horror I was living. I was done.

The vision of my wife and children coming down in the morning, finding me slumped over on the kitchen floor with my brains splattered all over the kitchen ceiling was the only thing that came to me then. Because I am one of those people who worship at the altar of science, I am a doubting Thomas about the existence of a Higher Power. But for whatever reason, and, again, it must have been Providence, I just put the gun down.

I started wailing like an injured animal because I was an injured animal. This was the most heart-wrenching wailing, like I had never wailed before in my life, and my wife came down from upstairs.

I ended up in an inpatient treatment program that morning. It was there that I met the woman who became my therapist. She went on to become one of my dearest and best friends in life, among many other AA friends and people in the recovering community. They got me back in the program and actively involved in the Recovering Nurses Association. I started putting one foot in front of the other.

For my first four months, I was not fit to lay hands on patients, so I was on disability. Then, I went back to work as a PA in the addiction treatment community where everyone knew that I was recently in treatment, newly sober and that my first priority was just to maintain my sobriety.

From there I went back to work as a PA in the areas of trauma, cardiology and the emergency room. Fortunately, I had not created a paper path with the state, although if I would have been reported and gone into the Physician's Health Program, it would not have been the worst thing in the world.

After getting actively involved with the Certified Registered Nurse Anesthetists, I decided to go to nursing school while continuing to work as a PA. I later went on to work as a nurse in the shock trauma ICU. After six or seven years of sobriety, I looked into becoming a nurse practitioner. I flipped over to nurse anesthesia, however, because I knew a good number of nurse anesthetists, many of whom I had thrown in the back of my car to take off to treatment while I was doing interventional work for the CRNAs.

I think it was my Higher Power who led me to this path in nurse anesthesia, but it was with a lot of questioning and a lot of adult supervision because there was always the concern about the high rate of addiction in the anesthesia community. The exposure in anesthesia to rocket fuel rather than the middle of the road drugs like morphine and Dilaudid raised some questions about the risk. But folks reassured me that, provided I did what I was supposed to do and stayed well-anchored in the recovery community, this really wouldn't be an issue. I think, for the most part, they were right.

In 2004, when I was about seventeen years sober, after the new policy statement of the American Nurses Association on impaired nursing was introduced and approved, my back began hurting. I thought I had just twisted it when taking a poster down. I went home and went to bed, but in the middle of the night, I got up with this horrible burning sensation and urgency to urinate.

I went into the bathroom and got this horrendous pain with a lightning-like shock. The next thing I remember was waking up on the bathroom floor with my dog licking my face and my wife coming out of the bedroom because she had heard a thud.

My pulse was so slow that I couldn't put a single sentence together. My wife thought I had a stroke because I could barely mumble anything recognizable and called for an ambulance. By the time that fire rescue got me in the ambulance, I became able to answer some questions.

When I arrived at the ER, I was stiff like a board. I would not let anyone roll me or touch me due to the pain. I kept repeating that I am in recovery and that I can't have any narcotics. I was told they needed to get some x-rays and a CAT scan, but I kept insisting that, if they put in an IV, the only thing they could give me was some Toradol.

After the IV was in and I was given Toradol, all the nurses were smiling, smirking at me. I'm not getting it at all. When they finally took me to x-ray and tried to roll me onto the table, I screamed in sheer agony. The doctor said he understood that I didn't want to take any pain medication but that they really needed to get the films. It finally occurred to me that this situation was not in my control. So, I finally said "OK" and they gave me two milligrams of Dilaudid intramuscularly. They told me it would be OK.

I can honestly tell you that before that needle was out of my butt, I wanted another two milligrams. What went right through my head was that this is a freebie, and that this is real. So why not go for the whole ball of wax?

I truly believe that once the brain is pickled, the neuroplasticity of the brain has altered the brain's wiring. My wiring was a little to the left of midline to begin with, prior to my addiction. Once there was the exposure to drugs and alcohol, my brain really got rewired. It never will go back to that premorbid state.

Despite my best efforts, I knew right then and there that the disease of addiction was alive and well in me. I was given a prescription for Percocet before I left the hospital but because I have a deal with my addictionologist that I would only take narcotics while in an inpatient setting under his supervision, I tore up the script when I got home.

I am NOT saying any other addict should do that, but I was so in awe of the malignancy and pervasiveness of my disease. I hobbled into work the next day because I knew once my chairman saw how much agony I was in, he would send me right in for an MRI. I got an MRI emergently at work, and then went to see my addictionologist, who arranged an EMG. After that, I was actually able to get the pain down to a dull roar.

My pain remains well-controlled today with the use of acetaminophen and non-steroidal anti-inflammatory medications. I do not support the use of opioid or any other abuse-able medications, except in addictionologist supervised emergencies. That means no opiates, no tramadol, no benzodiazepines. NONE!

Although my own recovery did not include the use of naltrexone, many CRNAs have experienced success with its use. Having one hundred percent mu receptor antagonist properties, naltrexone does not have the opioid agonist effects nor does it have any of the withdrawal phenomena associated with buprenorphine or methadone. So, while I am in full support of naltrexone where supervised appropriately by an addictionologist, I do not support the use of buprenorphine or methadone.

I have reaped incredible gifts for the past twenty-two years that are just beyond my wildest dreams. I mean, I never, ever thought I'd live to see thirty and then, once in my thirties, never thought I would live to reach forty. The concept that I would be sober now longer than I drank and drugged was certainly never a thought that percolated through my addicted head.

Burned All My Bridges To Recover

Even though I was not able to acknowledge or accept it early-on, my story of addiction started long before I became a nurse. Coming from a big family riddled with addiction, mostly alcoholism, I had a problem with alcohol before I ever started using drugs. I was into illegal drugs, mostly cocaine, pills and marijuana, prior to nursing school.

I was a single mother of two sons, on public assistance who knew that I needed to find a better life because I was living a life I didn't want for myself. The type of life I had was definitely not the life I wanted for my kids.

A public initiative was started back in 1988 to make people either work for their grants or go to school to get a trade. So, when I was offered an opportunity through the Department of Social Services to take part in their Welfare To Workfare program, I took it.

Since the time I had been a little girl, I had always wanted to be a nurse. Part of the reason was because my godmother was a nurse. She used to talk about how much she loved being able to help people and take care of them. I always had that type of personality, even though I didn't know how to take care of me back then. So, I figured if I was offered training to become a nurse, it would be my opportunity, my ticket out, so to speak.

So, I went down to the Department of Social Services to find out if nursing school was being offered and discovered that an LPN program was a possible option. After taking all the necessary preliminary tests, I was informed that nursing would be a good fit for me as I had scored high in math and sciences.

As time went on, I just knew I had to get through nursing school. Getting my nursing license was going to eventually give me my way out and be the thing that saved my life. Really, truly, it was.

At that time, the Welfare To Workfare program really took care of everything for me, except the studying. They picked me up in the morning, took me to school as well as the clinical setting and made arrangements for my children to attend daycare. Whatever I needed, they made sure that I got it. Basically, all I had to do was get out of bed in the morning and get myself and the kids ready and dressed. Except for doing the required course work and studying, everything else was taken care of.

While I was a pretty good student, I was definitely not living a lifestyle that was conducive to being a nursing student at the time. Although I know for sure that I started school the day that my youngest son turned six months old, my addiction was so bad at that point in my life that I can't remember a lot of things regarding my schooling,

After nursing school, I started my first nursing job as a graduate LPN, or GPN, in a nursing home. I passed my nursing board exams, was able to get my license and loved my job, but I still had an awful addiction.

About eight months on the job, my attendance became very poor due to my drug use. I was written up for my lateness and absence on a couple of occasions. Actually, the only reason I made it out of the house to go to work at all was because I needed to pay the rent to have a place to live.

Eventually, it got to the point where I couldn't get out of the house to go in to work anymore. My addiction had gotten so bad because I had started using cocaine and crack. At times, my paranoia was so great that I couldn't even leave my house. Some days I don't know how my older son even made it to school.

A prisoner in my own home, once I got high I couldn't leave the house. I lived two lives: the one outside the home, where it looked like there was nothing wrong, like my children and I were the All-American family; and the other, inside the home, which was a totally different story; a living nightmare.

The people I hung out with were not people that normal people would ever associate with. For lack of a better way to put it, I hung out with street people who had the same addiction problem I had. In essence, I was one of these street people, maybe only a little bit better off because I was a nurse with a respectable job. Yet I was living this horrendous lie.

One day, after having been up all night getting high, I got ready for work in the wee hours of the morning. I took my shower, ironed my uniform and walked to work. Mid-morning that day, I was passing medications. I don't know if I blacked out or fell asleep while standing up, but when I came to, I realized that the medication in the cup in front of me was not the medication for the patient I was about to dispense it to.

Extremely scared by this event, I knew I was in serious trouble with my addiction problem. If I was ever to hurt a patient by giving them the wrong medication, that would have been just awful. But while I was scared to death, I tried to justify what had happened because the meds in the cup were mostly

31

vitamins and stools softeners that wouldn't have hurt the patient. Inside, though, I knew it could have been devastating to the patient and their family if I had ever given the wrong medication out to anyone.

Realizing the seriousness of what might have happened due to my addiction, I finished working that day and I never went back to the nursing home. I knew at that point I had to do something. Basically, I had abandoned my job. I just did not know how to get better because once I started to get high on any given day I didn't know how to stop.

Getting high was all I knew. I did not know how not to get high. Living in an area where getting high was literally all everybody ever did, people used to come to my house at all hours of the day and night. It really was not a home I lived in but a drug den. Every day when I woke up, I felt the horrible cycle of guilt and shame. It was like being in my own hell. In order to not feel that pain anymore, I had to get high.

It got to a point where I couldn't make a simple decision like going to the deli across the street. I wasn't mentally there for my kids who were really captives in the house. Once Mommy got high, God forbid one of the neighbors talked to them while they were out playing. I was afraid neighbors would find out about what was going on in the house.

Although I don't remember doing anything drug-related in front of my kids, they knew what was going on. Drugs were so accepted and ever-present in the house that when there was a discussion in my son's school about drugs, he innocently blurted out in class, "Yeah, my Mom smokes crack." Needless to say, Child Protective Services came to my house that night to check, although the children were not taken out of the home.

Even though my family is relatively close, I wouldn't contact my family at all when I wasn't doing well. My brother became concerned when he hadn't heard from me for a few months after I had abandoned my job, so he came to see me.

Hearing a knock at the door, I looked out the window, saw him, went downstairs and invited him in. I remember I had to move a pile of dirty dishes and other things out of the way just so he could sit down at the kitchen table. There was a random person sleeping on the couch at the time and my younger son was home with me. My older son loved to go to school which was his escape. Although he missed school at times due to my irresponsibility when there were no clean clothes available for him to wear, he had made it to school that day particular day.

When I saw my brother looking around at the condition of my apartment, I told him that I was on vacation from my job and that we had a party last night in my house. A little further into his visit, I realized that there was no way my brother believed that excuse, because I didn't even believe what I said. So I told him that I was on drugs and needed help. I knew that things had gotten increasingly dangerous in my house because of the illegal drugs. The people I was now associating with were much worse than previously and my life was just a mess. So, in my heart, I knew that if I didn't get help I was going to die or, even worse, that something horrible was going to happen to my children.

For a couple of hours, my brother and I talked. I told him that I was thinking about going into a treatment program I had heard about. So, we got my younger son dressed, picked my older son up from school and went to my brother's house to call different treatment facilities.

Initially, I lied to my brother, telling him that I actually had an appointment at a facility. I lied to set his mind at ease, so he wouldn't worry about me. I also lied because I wanted more time to make the decision to fully commit myself to treatment. I was so scared to go into treatment since I had failed before. In fact, I had not even been able to stay to complete treatment in the past. I also had to consider who was going to care for my children while I was in treatment, but knew that since I had told my brother that I needed help, my family wasn't going to let me not get help, especially since my kids were in danger every day.

Finally, I contacted a treatment program and made an appointment for an intake on September 25th, 1991. Having been in treatment before and knowing where my addiction had taken me, I knew if I left my children with my family that they would have to give my children back to me even if I left treatment early. Since I did not want to have an excuse that would allow me to leave treatment prior to completion, even though my family offered to take care of my kids while I went to long-term treatment, I burned all my bridges. I got the legal system involved, so I basically forced my own hand to do the right thing and ensure that I completed treatment.

Through discussions with my family, we decided that the best thing for me to do was to put my kids into foster care. While I'll never know why CPS hadn't taken my kids from me the night they came to my house, I brought my children to the Department of Social Services with my Dad on September 26,

1991. I had talked to my kids a couple times prior to that day about where I was going. I told them that I would be getting the help I needed. My sons were very happy that I wasn't going to be sick or crazy or hiding anymore. I told them they were going to have a mother who was going to learn how to keep the promises she made to them, like going to the park to play with them. In the past, I had told my kids every day that I would take them to the park, but we never made it because I couldn't even make it out the front door.

I remember the DSS building was actually set down low, below the level of the street and parking lot. It seemed like it was in a valley and had several flights of stairs down to where the entrance was. I told Child Protective Services that I didn't have any family to care for my children. I wrote up a statement saying I was unable to take care of my children because I was an addict. I remember I also had to write that my children were in danger if they continued to live with me.

Saying goodbye to my sons who were three and six at the time was the hardest thing I had to do in my whole life, up until that point. The walk back up those stairs was endless. I never saw so many flights of steps in front of me before but I knew my sons were in a safer, better place.

Since I had admitted I was an active addict, I had to have supervised visits with my children in the beginning. In order to visit them, I had to go down to DSS for scheduled appointments. If there wasn't anything else I did in any given week, I made sure that I kept those appointments to visit with my kids. I wasn't yet able to get into treatment and was still using, but I knew I couldn't get high the night before visitation or the day I visited them. Religiously, I kept those appointments every week until I got into the treatment program.

Before this time, I had never actually acknowledged that I had a problem. I had heard stories about therapeutic communities being a nightmare and had already been through other treatment programs that, for whatever reason, were definitely not for me. Most of the time I had gone into treatment, it was for my Dad or just to shut somebody up or satisfy the minor legal problems I had gotten into as a kid.

Since the therapeutic community had no beds, I had to call every day at nine o'clock in the morning. I had been instructed that if I missed calling even one morning that they would assume I didn't want treatment and put my name at the end of the list. So, every day I called. I even remember calling several times, crying, saying, "You have to get me off the streets because I'm going to die out here."

It was awful not knowing how not to get high. Though I did not want to get high anymore, I didn't want not to get high either. I would look at my kids and realize that this was definitely not what I wished for them. I thought about having worked so hard to become a nurse and the opportunities I had been given.

Finally on Nov 5th, 1991, I was told that a bed would be available for me the next day, which was my younger son's seventh birthday. I called my Dad and asked to spend the night at his house. He could not understand why I wanted to do that, but I explained that if I didn't stay there, I would probably get high that night and would not be able to leave my house in the morning to get to the treatment program.

So, I packed all my clothes into two black garbage bags. I took my nursing books from school and the cardboard envelope that held my nursing license, put it under my arm, and sat on my front stoop waiting for my father to pick me up. Everything else I left behind in the apartment, even the people still getting high. They had no idea that I was leaving because I hadn't told them anything. I just left.

On November 6th, 1991, when I walked into the therapeutic community, my whole life started to change. I knew I was safe. For the next fifteen-and-a-half months, I stayed in treatment. I met the nurse there who is one of the nicest human beings I have ever met. After I was there a couple days, I remember having a conversation with her and I told her that I wanted to work with her someday. I will never forget what she told me at the time: "Get your act together and anything is possible."

That was the beginning of my new life in recovery. I found that I didn't have to get high anymore. I found that I didn't have to struggle with that insanity and that pain. It was just kind of lifted from me. I began to believe that no matter what happened to me in this program and no matter what I was afraid of, none of that was anywhere near as bad as what I had been doing to myself on the outside, before I got there.

I found out a whole lot of things about myself. The program gave me a lot of tools to use and helped me find out who I really was and where I had been. I also started to identify where I was going and where I wanted to go in life. I was taught how to be the person I always wanted to be inside and I remain so very grateful for that program to this very day.

While in treatment, I was offered HIV testing. When my oldest son was about eighteen months old, I had started using intravenous drugs for a very short period of time. I had stopped using them because some of the people I was associated with who were also using IV drugs at the time began looking unhealthy. The scare about what was to later be called HIV had just started to be publicized. So, rather than not get high at all, I just stopped IV drug use after about eight months and smoked crack and sniffed cocaine.

About ten months into treatment, I finally decided that I should have an HIV test. I remember on August 27, 1992, I learned that my test came back positive. At that time, I just thought my life was over. I thought, here I am, finally getting my life together, just to turn around and die from something else. All I could think about was how I didn't want to have HIV. Although I momentarily had the idea that I should leave the program, that notion was followed immediately by the realistic consideration, "Where am I going to go, back to the street?" In spite of the terrible news that I was HIV positive, I found that I didn't want to get high anymore.

The treatment program sent me to a good doctor at the medical center who initially started me on AZT, which was the only medication available back then. Then, I started to fear that I couldn't be a nurse anymore because I had HIV. It took me a good while to realize that I had to be more afraid of the patients than the patients needed to be fearful of me. The program sent me for a lot of educational courses about the precautions I needed to take. I did a lot of research on my own about HIV and I found that I can still be a nurse doing all the things nurses do, but that I had to do things a little bit differently to protect myself and others so no one is put at risk.

38

Over time, I also realized that I didn't feel any different physically after I received the diagnosis than I did before that time. Now, nearly eighteen years later, I still don't feel any different physically.

The whole time I was in treatment, I picked my kids up for the weekends. Although they were in foster care, I had retained my parental rights. Throughout my entire fifteen-and-a-half months in treatment, my children came back to stay with me at the treatment program on weekends since I had no home to take them to. I remained actively involved with my children and interacted with their foster care worker regularly.

When I was getting ready to finish the treatment program, I went to the Director of Medical Services and asked if they had any jobs available for me. I told her I would really like to work for the treatment program because I truly believe in what the program has to offer people. The director told me that they didn't hire LPNs, but to give her some time to see what she could do. Ultimately, a position was created for me.

When I interviewed for the job, I told the director that she would not be sorry that she hired me. I said that I would do whatever they wanted me to do because I wanted to have a part in helping other people save their own lives. Like a partnership made in heaven, I worked alongside the same nurse who took care of me in treatment and had told me that anything was possible. At the time, she became my colleague and friend. Today, I still work for the program and she is my closest and best friend.

Upon completion of the treatment program, there was a tremendous ceremony with a big reception, similar to a prom or a wedding. Graduates could bring two family members or friends to the sit-down dinner which included a dance. I remember the day we were rehearsing for our graduation ceremony because my kids were still in foster care. My older son had been pretty ill on and off for months. He would seem to get better and then he would be sick again. The doctors couldn't figure out what was going on with him. Each time he was treated, the social worker needed to get my permission, so I went to the medical appointments.

At this particular appointment shortly before graduation, I called the doctor aside, told him my son had been sick for a-while now and did not seem to be getting better. I disclosed to the doctor that I was HIV positive and asked if that could have anything to do with why my son wasn't getting any better. The doctor said he didn't know but that my HIV status probably had nothing to do with his illness. He put my son on an antibiotic and sent us home.

When we left, I called the director who had hired me. I asked her if my son could be tested for HIV at the treatment program because the doctors couldn't find out what's wrong with him. I called my foster care worker, told her the situation and that I was going to take my older son back to the program with me to have him tested. Since my younger son was healthy, I did not ask to have him tested and only took my older son back to the program with me for the test.

A couple of weeks later I learned that my nine year-old was infected. At that point, I knew I didn't want him back in foster care because I didn't know how much information the foster care worker was going to tell the foster parents. I didn't know how much any of them knew about HIV and did not want my children to be hurt or stigmatized because of that. So I called the doctor specializing in HIV who had been treating me since I was diagnosed and asked if she would see my son. Since she didn't treat children, she referred him to another doctor and I got an appointment to bring both my sons in the very next day.

I called foster care and told her I would keep the kids overnight, since at that point it was just a matter of time before I would take my kids back permanently. By this time, I had my own apartment in preparation for graduation from treatment and was just waiting to have day care in place before my sons came back to live with me.

When I went to the doctor the next day with my sons, there was a great team of HIV specialists who just scooped my children up. They took both kids in like they were their very own children. My older son was found to have pneumonia.

As several appointments were scheduled after that, I called the foster care worker and told her I would be keeping the kids. While she initially said, "You can't do that," I insisted, telling her that I needed to do whatever it took to make sure that my children got the very best medical care possible. The foster care worker accepted that and made the necessary arrangements, so from that day on I actually kept my sons.

In the beginning, it was a pretty rocky road. My sons were used to the old me, the Mom who used drugs. Time passed and in 1996, my older son started getting sick a lot. He would get terrible sinus infections repeatedly. A PIC line was inserted and he was treated at home for infections on a long-term basis.

I asked a social worker at my job who worked with clients with HIV to tell my son his diagnosis. I didn't know how I would handle it if my son looked up at me and asked me if he was going to die. I knew I wasn't going to be able to handle something like that, so the social workers took him out a couple of times, did some counseling with him and told him his diagnosis.

My son handled his diagnosis much differently than I handled mine. If it was appropriate to the conversation, I would pretty much tell anybody and, on occasions, even used my diagnosis as a learning tool with clients at work. On the other hand, my son kept his diagnosis to himself and would not disclose it to anyone, which was his right, out of fear that his friends would not like him or understand.

Our differences in handling our diagnoses worked out very well because I respected his wishes. There were some issues with his school a couple times because I did make the school aware that he was HIV infected. One issue arose when my son had a cold and sneezed in school. The principal called and told me I had to pick him up because he spit on the floor. It wasn't a matter of him spitting but some mucous came out of his nose when he sneezed. Everyone became hysterical at the time and the principal wanted to suspend him. After that incident, we moved out of that school district to have a much better experience in his next school.

For about three years, my son's condition was up and down. My son was in pretty bad shape towards the end of 1996, when protease inhibitors were approved for adults. I remember talking to his doctor about the possibility of him being placed on them, but she said there was really no information on dosing kids and the medications were very toxic. Because of all the antibiotics he had been on in the past, my son's liver was not very healthy to begin with.

Over time, my son got very, very sick and stopped taking his medication. I used to find pills stashed everywhere; under the chair table legs, pushed down into the carpet. His pills would be all lined up in the little baseboard radiator shutters. It was really like an Easter egg hunt when I went looking for his medication.

In February of 1997, it was very apparent that my son wasn't doing well. I realized that he wasn't going to get any better. My son realized this, too, and he had been out of school since November the year before because of his PIC line.

My son had stopped eating, not because he didn't want to eat but because he couldn't digest anything. The only thing he could tolerate was this awful iced tea. He used to live on that and I would mix pitchers and pitchers of it for him. Every once in awhile, he would tell me he wanted to eat a T-bone steak. He'd say, "Mom, I want a steak." He would eat the whole steak but then he wouldn't eat for weeks. I don't know where he put it, but he would devour that whole T-bone steak.

He had been an active little boy when he wasn't sick. Whatever was going on, he always had so much energy. He was totally all-boy. He loved to play football and baseball, went skateboarding and roller skating, and when he was twelve, he even started to like girls.

One day, though, when I looked at him, I saw that the whites of his eyes were glowing yellow. I happened to be at my job at the time and he was outside playing. When he came in, he seemed a little tired with his eyes just glowing yellow. I asked him if he could go to the bathroom and he gave me a urine specimen the color of coffee. When my son saw his urine, I think it frightened him because he told me that he thought an x-ray might help.

That was a Sunday and I called his doctor immediately. She said to bring him in the next day and my son asked to speak to the doctor. When my son told her he thought he needed an x-ray, she told him that when he came in to see her he could have whatever he wanted.

The next day, the doctor and I sat down and spoke while the social worker took my son down for the x-ray he wanted. The doctor told me that my son was in liver failure; that we would keep him as comfortable as possible for as long as possible, but that he wasn't going to get any better.

In the beginning of March, 1997, my son knew he wasn't going to get any better. He had overheard me on the phone with my Dad talking about the deed to a family cemetery plot where I wanted him buried next to my Mom.

When I got off the phone, my son asked me about it and we discussed it. Knowing it was just a matter of time, he helped me plan his funeral. There were a lot of things that he requested. He asked me if he could give a message to his classmates. Although he had tried to visit his classmates at lunchtime once awhile back when he was in a wheelchair, the principal thought that the visit might be too upsetting for the other kids.

The social worker who used to come by to visit my son had a long talk with him. They came to the conclusion that my son would make a videotape recording of himself that could be played for his classmates. So on March 17th, 1997, a journalist came to the house with another social worker and my son was interviewed on camera. They made this little video which was really an interview where my son answered their questions because he was pretty sick at that point.

Afterwards, my son watched the video. Then he asked me to request that the school play the video for his class, but made me promise that I would not do that until after he died. Of course, I told him I would do what he asked.

On the 25th of March, 1997, my son passed away at the age of twelve. It's funny that not once throughout this entire ordeal did I ever want to use. That was just not an option for me because I knew that it was not going to make anything better. Still, to this day, I don't ever want to use again because using never makes anything better. No matter what the situation may be, using just makes everything more chaotic, crazier, worse.

There was a documentary on HIV and AIDs made out of my son's little video. Since my son would be twenty-five years of age now, I have to be HIV infected for at least the past twenty-six years. Looking back, the HIV infection was caused by unprotected sex that I had before my son was born, since my IV drug use started when he was already a toddler.

A lot of good things have come out of my recovery. I have two wonderful jobs at two different drug treatment programs. I have the ability to use my story to help other people and to be an active participant in other people's recovery. I am able to let people know that no matter what you have to go through in life, you don't ever have to get high again. There is a much better way.

Sober since November 6th, 1991, my recovery remains strong today. I love being clean and sober. I love being a nurse and part of the treatment program that got me clean and sober. I think I have the best possible job in the world for someone like me.

I am very, very lucky that situations arose in my life as they did to help me to help myself be where I am today. In order to be where I am today in my recovery, I would not change anything that I have been through in life, other than my son being infected with HIV. I thank God that my younger son is not HIV positive. As long as I remain in recovery, I know that there is absolutely nothing in this world that I can't do.

I Love Who I Have Become

Now fifty-three years old, I am the oldest of three children of Polish and Lithuanian parents. My mother had three miscarriages before she delivered me, so I was that chosen child. My brother was born a year and a half later and my sister about a year after that. My father was a machinist.

My mother grew up in a home where she was the baby of an alcoholic dad. As a girl, she had to go to the bars to bring her father home for dinner. He would be singing at the top of his lungs as they walked through the streets on the way home, which was quite an embarrassment to her. The first time I remember hearing her talk about her father was when I came home drunk as a young teen. She said, "You're going to be just like my father." Ever since that time, she has denied he had a problem because he never missed a day of work as a tailor.

My father was from the Polish side of the family and had a twin brother. One of eight children, my father got the cat-and-nine-tails from his dad who was a drinker and liked to hit him with it. My dad has always been a quiet man, kind of sealed up. It's very hard to get him to talk.

We lived on the third floor of my mother's parents' house for the first four years of my life, so we had a lot of family support. When my parents bought a house and moved to the suburb, it was a big change for my mother because she didn't drive.

My parents struggled a lot financially because my dad went on strike a lot. During those periods there would be no money coming in, so my mother learned to be very frugal along the way because she had to. We weren't destitute poor, but we were poor. I wore hand-me-downs from my mother's friend's daughter.

I remember my father had some sort of head injury in the workplace and was out of work for six months. At the time, the doctors couldn't figure out what was going on with his injury and he wasn't getting paid. His side of the family did not do anything to support our family except that one of the aunts brought over a jar of peanut butter once. We were able to hang onto the house because my mother's father helped us out as best he could and my parents still live there, to this day.

After the head injury, nobody seemed to know what was happening with my dad. So when I heard some talk about his x-ray showing a brain tumor, I thought my dad was going to die. We didn't talk about it in my family because we didn't really talk about anything at home. I came to find out that this lack of communication was a very important part of my up-bringing.

Hugging and anything like that was not the norm in my house. We were not a touchy-feely kind of family. The only time I ever heard the word love being used was when I was being punished. My parents would say, "We're punishing you because we love you." It wasn't really good for me to connect the term love with punishment, but I did. Being poor, having an innate lack of self-esteem, and having nobody to talk to about my feelings, was a really shitty combination which was not the best for healthy child development.

So, with some good genetic material from two alcoholic grand-dads, parents who didn't talk and a sister who could be very nasty at times, it was tough growing up. I would not go back in time if I had the chance unless I could do so with the knowledge I have now. Knowledge like what to do with the feelings of inadequacy, or not being pretty enough, or smart enough.

Even though my sister and I get along better now, I remember being with two of my friends one day when she said we were all sluts. I went raging after her with a pair of scissors because I did not know how to verbally speak up about the feelings I had. While I still might get upset at times, I don't use scissors anymore. Back then, though, I stuffed all the negative feelings within me until I had an outburst of rage.

As a teenager, I wasn't the jock, or the cheerleader, or the smart kid, so I connected with the druggies in high school. I did a lot of experimenting, met a lot of cool people and did a lot of fun things like sitting in the woods, tripping.

When I graduated from high school, I went to a three-year nursing school. That's where I met two friends who lived with me in the dorm for three years. The first year we got to stay in the nursing school dorm over the weekends, so we went to the clubs and partied. We became groupies with a band that had good drugs and a lot of alcohol.

I was looking for love in all the wrong places and trying to make some sort of a connection when I didn't really have a connection with myself. I was sexually active because I wanted somebody to love me and help me feel good. So, at the time, my life was sex, drugs and rock-n-roll, and I did the gamut of them.

Although I did not apply myself very much back then I managed to graduate from nursing school. I got a job and stayed

49

at a girlfriend's house. We were all going to this bar and that's where I met some new friends, including a man I later married.

One night, I went into the city with my friends, smoked a lot of weed and drank a lot of wine. Although I had driven under the influence before without consequences, after driving my friend to her boyfriend's house, I passed out at the wheel of my little convertible about twenty minutes from where I was going. The memory is still so clear because I remember that I came to with the car tipped at an embankment. My car had knocked down all these little trees.

I must have passed out again because when I woke up, I was outside the car, face down in the dirt. My eight track cassette was still playing music because the car was still running. Re-calling movie scenes where cars exploded after crashes, I tried to get up, even though my leg felt kind of funny. I didn't look at my leg and hobbled down to the side of the road to get someone to stop.

After a few cars passed, a nurse and her boyfriend stopped. She was really good, with a calming presence, and reassured me through this whole ordeal. As other cars showed up at the scene, I gave her my pocketbook because there was stuff in there that I didn't want the police to find.

The ambulance came and took me to the same hospital where I worked nights. Later on, I heard from a supervisor that I was cursing up a storm on admission. I went to surgery the next day for cleaning of my leg wound. I actually had a huge flap hanging off the back of my leg which required two more sur-geries, including a skin graft.

While at the hospital, this guy from the bar came to visit me a lot. He used to bring me Riuniti Rosato wine and we would mix it with Seven-Up. So I had these little wine spritzers which were especially fabulous to drink with my pain medication on top of them.

The little relationship with this guy started during my hospital stay, but something else started, too. I got my very first taste of Percocet. I remember the minute I swallowed those first little pills, something changed for me. It was like heaven on earth. I felt so OK with myself; like I finally found the place where I most wanted to be in the world.

Very comfortable in the hospital with my Riuniti and pain medication, I started my incredible run, looking for medications out there. My leg was so mangled up and I was feeling really awful about myself. I remember telling the nursing supervisor that I would never be able to wear a dress again, feeling so depressed with this big crater in the back of my knee. I felt everyone was looking at it, which just added to the lack of good feelings I already had about myself, so I was on the hunt for more drugs to cope with that.

Out of the hospital, this guy and I became an item and married in 1981. The relationship started out great because he was in the bar industry and we would drink a lot. He had connections with people who knew people who robbed drug stores and so I got myself a BIG bottle of Percodan. I was eating them like candy because I liked the way they made me feel.

Back to working nights, I was looking for something in one of the patient's medication drawers and found some Tylenol with codeine. Since it was not counted back then, I decided to try those for some residual back pain from the accident one night.

The Tylenol with codeine gave me a somewhat similar feeling to the one I had when I was first given Percocet. My diversion of the easy-to-get meds in patient's drawers, like Tylenol #3 and Talwin, started at that point.

After awhile, I escalated to diverting the controlled meds like Percocet from the narcotic cabinet. The hospital must have been watching me for awhile because one night they floated me to a day surgery floor where patients spent the night before going home. One nurse would usually give the medications on that unit, so the hospital was able to hone in on me to make sure I was the one stealing the medications.

Sometime after working that shift, I got called into the nursing director's office on my day off. My husband drove me in because I didn't have a good feeling about it. The Director of Nursing, pharmacist and supervisor confronted me with the narcotic sheets. The pharmacist pointed out that all the Tylenol #3 was gone and yet there were not many patients documented as receiving any. So, I finally admitted to taking the Tylenol #3, but denied the Percocet diversion.

Terminated from employment and terribly upset, I left the hospital. My husband was waiting outside and just said, "Don't worry. You'll get another job. You'll be fine." There was never any talk about addiction or problems and we just kept plowing through.

So, I got a job on the night shift at another facility, being in charge of the medications and the patients. My former employer had not reported me to the Board of Nursing because that wasn't done much back then. At the time, I didn't even have a clue that I had committed a felony. I don't know what I was thinking, but it wasn't anything along those lines.

I went to work, listened to report, went through all the charts and gathered all the information on my patients. Even though I had told myself I would never steal drugs at the new job, the whole time I was listening to report and going through charts, I was just dying to get in there to pour those meds. I tried really hard not to take anything, but once I started obsessing about those pills, I could not help myself. I just had to have them. Once they were in my possession, I would somehow start to feel better.

I have read that this happens with other nurses, too. The minute the meds are in your hand, you don't even have to ingest them before being flooded with that sense of relief. That happened to me all the time, like clockwork. I would experience that incredible, insatiable need to find and get my source. So, I would get the medications, put them on the med tray, take the whole tray into the bathroom with me and do my thing. That long road downhill began and I went down it very fast.

The drugs by mouth stopped working, of course, so I took a big step over to Demerol. I brought my first dose home and shared it with my husband. We both had intramuscular injections of Demerol and it was a horrible experience for me. I became extremely itchy and started scratching like crazy. Although I never wanted to use Demerol again, I wasn't ready to stop taking drugs, so I moved on to morphine, and later Dilaudid, always intramuscularly, never intravenously.

Making sure I covered my diversion in the charting was a lot of work. I would sign out that I took the medication from the narcotic box, but wouldn't sign that the patient got it. I had an elaborate system and sort of managed, for awhile, until I started needing more and more medication. With opiates you just

53

can't get enough, so you have to keep upping the ante which really began to take its toll on me.

Probably up to about twelve milligrams of Dilaudid intramuscularly towards the end, I would take some just after report at midnight. By four a.m., I needed more. Getting more was becoming difficult and I found it harder to cover my tracks with the documentation. I became scared that I might lose my nursing license and it was that fear which motivated me to start looking for help.

My first attempt at outpatient treatment was when I thumbed through the yellow pages for a counselor. That's just about what that PhD was worth because his response to my telling him what I was doing at work was, "Well, I want you to go into work tonight and not take anything." Obviously, he did not know much about addiction because if I could have done that I would never have called him.

My next attempt at treatment was more successful. I found a counseling agency that had recovering addicts working there. I was comfortable being there, even though my counselor was tough, to the point and set up toxicology screens. I would go in for my session, pee in a cup and then go to the water fountain to take my Percocet. I would then head out for the day, feeling energized and alive because I could get a lot of things done on Percocet. Taking Percocet also made me feel better about the lousy things going on in my life, like my husband's drinking and drugging.

I remember asking my therapist one day how my urine results were and he said they were all clean. When I later confessed to him that I was still using, he said, "Yeah, I know." Surprised by his answer, I asked how he knew. He said because there was nothing about me that had changed since I started treatment. To this day, his response is something I always pay attention to with my clients because when people are recovering, something changes in them. It's not just about going to meetings and doing X, Y and Z.

Since I realized outpatient treatment wasn't working for me, I made the decision to go into the hospital for inpatient treatment. When I told my job I was going to have some surgery to fix up my mangled leg, coworkers asked what hospital they could send cards to. I worked very hard to remain evasive, which was just another part of the huge amount of work this addict had to do. I finally managed to tell them to just send any cards to my home and went out on a leave of absence.

So, about six months after I'd gotten married, I was admitted to a little six bed inpatient unit. While there for five or six weeks, I put in my resignation because I knew I couldn't go back to where I was working. During my entire stay on the unit, I was the only female. I fell madly in love with one of the charmers there who was very bad news, although I never acted on any of my impulses with him. I was still feeling love starved, so I was looking for love in all the wrong places. I've since learned that love starts with me.

My family and my husband's parents visited me in treatment, but my husband never quite made it in to see me. There was a family meeting at one point with my parents, brother and sister to help us build communication skills. I remember my dad, who never said much, mentioned he sometimes doesn't feel loved by the family, and I jumped right in, saying, "How can you say that? Of course we love you!" The counselor just said, "Stop. It's a feeling he's having. Don't jump in and try

55

to alleviate his feelings." That was the first time I ever remember my dad talking about feelings he had inside.

Part of the inpatient treatment program was going to Alcoholics Anonymous meetings and I was given a weekend pass to identify meetings in my area I could attend after discharge. There were no Narcotics Anonymous meetings in my area at that time. I met a nurse at one of the meetings who agreed to be my temporary sponsor until I found a permanent one.

When I returned to the unit, I brought an old purse from home that I had not emptied of all its contents. When the staff checked it, they found some cocaine and a mirror which led them to suspect that I had used drugs on my pass. Although they threatened to kick me out, I really didn't want to go and was able to convince them to let me stay. I knew I was not ready to be out there on my own.

The pivotal point in treatment for me was when the night nurse read the poem "Footprints." The words made perfect sense to me at a time when I was struggling with the concept of a Higher Power. Suddenly, something clicked inside and I had a very powerful "Ah-Hah" moment. I was able to get myself a Higher Power and began feeling that I was not alone from that point on.

After discharge, I literally had to plan my entire day around meetings. Every day, I went to meetings, which became my new drug of choice. I got involved in the grassroots efforts which firmly established the NA program in my state. The meetings were very intimate back then and everyone knew everyone else.

NA became my everything. I met other recovering people there who were struggling like me. Because I had a car, and many others didn't, I became the one who drove others to meetings. This was wonderful because it made me get in my car and go to a meeting. Being responsible for taking others to meetings was a good way to make sure I went to a meeting, especially when I did not feel like going to one.

Looking back, we often went out for coffee after a meeting. This was a fabulous time in my life; a very social period where I felt alive, like I was shining and on top. This started my healing process. I once felt dead inside, but now there was a flicker of HOPE.

Instead of getting a job in nursing, I got a job working in a flower shop for that first year, even though my license was active. I needed a place to work that would not interfere with my getting to meetings. I also started going to Al Anon, which was really good for me, because my husband was still an obnoxious drunk. While I tried not to make any big changes that first year in recovery like the program suggests, his drinking was annoying the shit out of me.

Here I was, getting up every day and going to work, only to see him passed out at the wheel of the car in front of the house with his beer bottle between his legs. The first time I saw him like that, his window was open because it was summer. I punched him, yelled at him and went off to work. The second time I saw him like that, I wailed on him and went on my way to work. The third time I saw him, I walked right on by. I was getting healthier.

Even though I was dealing with the situation better because of Al Anon, we had a final episode which proved to be the turning point in our marriage. One night, when arguing in the kitchen, I picked up a knife and was going to stab that son-of-a-gun. There but for the grace of God, what went through my mind at that moment was that if I killed him, I would go to jail and I hadn't just done all this hard work in recovery to go off to jail.

So, I put the knife down, called my sponsor, left the house and never went back again. I stayed with my sponsor for three or four weeks, sleeping on the floor of her apartment. I continued going to meetings, working in the flower shop and found a new place to live.

Although my husband and I went for some couples counseling, we got a divorce. He didn't see he had a problem with alcohol and I recognized I had made a mistake marrying him. I also began to understand why I had married him. He was gregarious, outgoing and could talk to anyone, yet I used to need drugs to talk to people. I thought I could get his traits through osmosis.

I kept a sponsor for a while and at one point ended up meeting my sponsor's sister. I had become very concerned about my sponsor because she was a manic depressive who was losing jobs and had stopped her medication. I told her sister and we did an intervention on my sponsor together. This was a very tough thing for me to do. I expressed my concern and love for my sponsor but told her if she didn't take her meds I could not chose to be in her life.

The intervention didn't go so well because my sponsor got very angry. While I stopped having her as a sponsor, her sister and I bonded like magnets and became very good friends. After that, I never really had a sponsor, but I always had lots of people I could talk to about feelings. I started to form the types of relationships where people would help me if I needed it. Not all of these people were in recovery, but I did not hang out with people who drank or used drugs. I was making much better choices about the people around me and noticed that, as I got better, the people around me were getting better.

Still not very self-confident, I got involved in doing NA service. I started a meeting on Monday nights and truly felt like I really belonged. I offered to be the group treasurer. Everyone seemed very comfortable with that, although looking back their comfort may have been because I was one of the few in the group who had a car and a paycheck at the time.

After a full year at the flower shop, I began looking for a job in nursing and got a full-time position doing IV therapy. This meant I didn't have to be around the narcotic box. While my entire social life at the time revolved around NA, I never told anyone on the IV team that I was an addict in recovery because I was afraid they wouldn't trust me and would lock up their money.

One day, I finally took the plunge and told one of the nurses I worked with that I'm an addict in recovery who goes to NA meetings. She thought that was great and told me her uncle was in recovery from alcoholism. When I told her that I had thought if she knew of my history she would be afraid of me and hide her purse, she just said, "Oh, geez." This experience showed me it was OK to talk about recovery with my co-workers because it was accepted. It was a really big turning point for me because it was the first time I had told a non-recovering person what I was all about.

Being more open about my recovery opened the door for me to get a job after working on the IV team for four years. So in 1985, I began working at a treatment facility helping impaired health professionals. When I moved quite a distance from the facility and the commute became unbearable, I got a position providing Employee Assistance Services to impaired nurses in 1989. For the next twenty years, until I retired in 2009, I did the initial assessments and treatment referrals as well as the intensive follow-up these very complex EAP cases involving impaired nurses required.

Over the years, and especially after I moved from the area I originally got sober in, my meeting attendance started to drop. Trying to establish and develop a new life here, I found the meetings were not like they were back home. NA had grown as a program, so the size of the meetings was overwhelming compared to the intimate groups where everyone used to know everyone else.

Although some people say that people who stop going to meetings don't hear about what happens to people who stop going to meetings and then relapse, it is not as simple as that. Over the years I have been in recovery, I haven't been just going to NA meetings. My recovery expanded and included strong relationships where I talk intimately to my close friends and periodically go to therapy, as situations arise. Basically, I have been expunging all the toxins I had within me since entering recovery in 1982.

While my meeting attendance may have dwindled, I kept going to the NA conventions, and maintained many friendships in the program. I have also kept up with my connections back where my recovery started. I still get down on my knees every day to ask my Higher Power to keep me away from any drugs and for the knowledge of His will for me and the power to carry it out. By doing this, I have made room for healthy people and activities to come into my life.

For a long time in recovery, I lived by myself and focused on my recovery. Sixteen years ago, I married a very insightful man who is my very best friend. I trust him fully. He is not afraid to give me feedback on what he sees going on with me. It takes a special someone, who loves me a lot, to tell me things I probably don't want to, but need to, hear. I cannot make changes if I don't think anything needs changing. It's painful to hear some things, but I know that he is speaking to me through his heart.

We have a child who brought a huge change to our relationship when we adopted him at seventeen months old. It's strenuous work having a thirteen year old son who has Asperger's syndrome. Some of what he says and does triggers the abuse I took from other kids when I was growing up. Since there is no end to the changes in life, we are back in therapy with a professional who knows Asperger's syndrome, which is truly a God-send.

I hang out with a group of wonderful women who are really lovely people. We have our regular "girl's nights out." We go out to dinner and the theater. We talk a lot, and the more we talk, the less we feel alone with our issues. I feel so much a part of this circle of women and know that they love me. So when my son says I'm boring or no fun, I can say, "Believe it or not, I have friends who think I am funny and just LOVE being with me!"

Sometimes I don't feel totally self-confident, especially if I think people seem to be looking at me in public. It's like an old tape flashing up, "Why are they looking at me? What's wrong with me?" Thank God, I am free of that most of the time now and I credit some of the improvement to EMDR, Eye Movement Desensitization Reprocessing. It has helped me think about traumatic situations today without all my past shame-based feelings.

Sober since February 1st, 1982, I see myself now as someone who initially got off track, but who developed all the potential they had been given at birth. I was born into my situation, and have been picking up valuable tools along the way to create the person I have become. I am so very grateful that my disease of addiction was identified and that treatment was available. I am GLAD I'm a recovering addict, because I love who I've become.

I Kept Coming Back

I'm a forty-three year old nurse who has remained sober since December 19th of 1987. Over the years, I have addressed many other addictions. After smoking three packs of cigarettes a day, I stopped smoking sixteen years ago. I've attended Overeaters Anonymous meetings since 1987, and although I have only had success staying abstinent for the last four years, I "kept coming back."

Finally debt-free after attending Debtors Anonymous, my life is working for me, instead of me working to pay my credit cards. I have spent time in Al-Anon and currently attend two fellowships regularly: OA and AA. My life is good today and I want to keep it that way. That's why I go to meetings! Recovery has been a process for me and still is.

My history, like that of many others with a history of addiction, is complicated and painful. It took time for me to put the pieces of the puzzle together as to how my childhood was still interfering with my adulthood. My family history is important as I need to see the big picture of where I came from.

I know very little about my parents who were from Ireland. They didn't speak much about where they came from. They were late bloomers who started their family after the age of forty. I am the youngest of their six children.

My mother was raised in a convent after her mother died. There was a priest in her family as well as the disease of alcoholism. My mother was well-educated, with a sense of arrogance about her. Stern, proper and disciplined, like a nun, there was little nurturing from her. I loved her, although she was untouchable to me.

My father was one of the oldest of twelve children. His father was a postman who was a severe alcoholic. When my father grew up, it was acceptable for children to be beaten by those who had authority over them. Being no exception, my father told me of the time his father had broken his appendix after the schoolmaster had beaten him.

A broken boy who went on to be a broken man from a broken home and country, my father went to work every day as a skilled union carpenter. Softer than my mother, he fed the homeless and went to church. There were parts of him that were good and, in spite of the twinkle in his eye, parts of him that were really evil and twisted; a direct result of his up-bringing.

Until about five years ago, I didn't remember most of my childhood because it was so horrible. I dealt with all my problems and traumatic upbringing through drug use, alcohol abuse, food, smoking and spending. Basically, all I knew how to do was run from my feelings.

My father snuck alcohol behind my mother's back and gave me my first drink when I was under the age of ten. Although he told me it wouldn't hurt me, he also told me not to tell my mother. My family was full of secrets and, to this day, still is.

So, I started drinking and running around the streets at the age of eleven. The first time I came home drunk, I had urine all over myself. My sister and mother hit me and let me sleep in my own vomit to teach me a lesson. Although the smell of vomit stayed in my mattress for years, I kept drinking because alcohol gave me the numb I was looking for.

While attending a private Catholic high school, there wasn't a single day that I didn't use something to "get out of myself."

Anorexic by sixteen, I was addicted to diet pills. My weight dropped to as low as eighty-five pounds and I hated myself and my body.

Looking back, I can see how the alcohol and the food addiction distracted me in many ways. Those addictions kept me alive at the time by numbing all the traumatic, painful feelings I had inside. Even so, I remember I had to talk myself out of killing myself on a daily basis on the way to high school on the train.

At eighteen, I packed two shopping bags filled with my belongings and left home. I worked three jobs to pay the rent to sleep on someone's couch. Book-smart and at the top of my class, I wanted to go to college, but I had to turn down the scholarships I received because I had no home to live in.

After I left home, no one in my family spoke to me. If you didn't do it my family's way, which was to go to college or get married, you were cut off. It was as if I didn't exist and I decided to move out west to get farther away from them.

The loneliness was incredible when I left home as a young girl. I wasn't that social and was very alone. When my girl-friends went out to go dancing and looking for guys, I went out to get drunk. I had many blackouts and, at times, became violent because the alcohol opened up the rage I felt inside. I drove drunk on many occasions and I thank God that I never hurt anyone.

Working in a business where there was a lot of drinking and cocaine, I had many drinking buddies. After a while, though, no one wanted me around because I was a lush and sloppy. I got addicted to cocaine, which cleaned up my drinking for awhile, but wiped out my money and dignity.

I didn't really know exactly what I was running from because my memories were still buried, but I was running fast. Becoming more isolated, my drinking got worse. I couldn't get enough. At the end of my drinking, I was drinking alone at home and hearing voices. I was only twenty-one and scared.

At that time, I worked with a man who was in Gamblers Anonymous. He was very honest with me, told me I was a mess and introduced me to Alcoholics Anonymous in 1987. That's when I began going to meetings and got sober. I had no idea what the sign "But for the Grace of God" on the wall at the meetings meant, but I sensed a genuine caring from the women at my very first meeting. That is what kept me coming back.

Shortly after I stopped drinking, I suffered a major nervous breakdown. Without the alcohol and drugs to suppress all my memories, they began coming up. While I didn't relapse, I spent several months locked up in a mental hospital on a MICA unit for mentally ill chemically addicted clients. I remember being abused by other patients while there and at one point had my head stuffed in a toilet. Going to AA meetings in the hospital was what helped me to connect with people who weren't labeled "insane."

Before the age of twenty-three, I went on to have several other nervous breakdowns due to the old trauma that was inside of me. Diagnosed with bipolar disorder, I was put on the mood stabilizer, lithium. That was many years ago when being on medication in AA was considered a very shameful thing. There are still many opinions out there today about being on medication but I am no longer embarrassed about it. I know where I come from; why I have a mood disorder; and for over twenty years have remained emotionally stable with no further hospitalizations.

Life was OK during my first ten years of recovery in AA but I was eating compulsively. I was also in and out of destructive relationships. Looking back, I wasn't very nice or kind to myself. While I had a very good job and the outside looked good, my insides were a wreck. Anxiety started to take over. My father died, I was laid off from my wonderful job and my life began to unravel.

Since everyone had always told me that I looked like a nurse, I decided to go to nursing school. As a perfectionist, I did very well in school. I studied hard and was recognized as being the kindest, most compassionate nursing student in my class. Ironically, by the time I graduated the nursing program at the age of thirty-two, I was so fearful of being trapped that I couldn't even get into the elevator at the hospital to see my patients. While everyone thought I was just being healthy taking the stairs, I was spending so much energy just trying to cover up my anxiety. Pretending I was OK, I was able to stay sober, but the food was increasingly out of control.

In my early thirties, I met a very handsome marine. He was a very angry man but I was used to angry men. He was also very abusive, which was all I knew from childhood, and all I thought I deserved. Early in the relationship, he told me that he had been in prison for raping a thirteen year-old girl. He said he really didn't do it; that the sex was consensual; that she was a "loose girl."

Feeling terrible for him having spent time in prison as an innocent man, I went ahead and married him. I was so far away from even loving myself at the time that I didn't know what love was. It wasn't until years later in my recovery that I realized that I was not only attached to abusers but also felt responsible for protecting them.

At thirty-five, I gave birth to my daughter; the light of my life. Born very sick and premature with many complications, I promised God that if he left her here with me on earth that I would do my very best to take care of her. And He did. At two months of age, I brought her home from the hospital and quit my job to take care of her full-time.

Meanwhile, my husband was becoming increasingly violent and abusive. It was a very difficult time during which I went to nine different therapists trying to get my husband fixed. Today, I know I should have just looked deeply at myself and fixed me, but I wasn't able to do that at the time.

Even though he was violent towards me, I never thought he would hurt my daughter. I was wrong. When she was only two, he smacked her in the face in front of me to provoke me. Later on, I found out that he had also choked her and hit her. So I began living with bags of clothes, diapers and baby bottles in the trunk of my car because at any moment I'd have to pick up and spend the night at a friend's house.

Finally, I found a wonderful therapist who began to work with me and I left the marriage. The night he kicked my daughter's crib while I clutched her in my arms, I told myself, "That's it. My daughter is not going to have the life that I had." I remember hiding from him on the floor under the couch because I knew he had a gun. I left the house with my daughter in my arms and her heart medication in my hand.

Now about seventeen years sober, my weight was close to two hundred pounds. My panic attacks were just brutal, often waking me in the middle of the night. I couldn't tolerate the

68

anxiety anymore but didn't want to go on medication for anxiety. I was always going to healing masses, trying to find some kind of help.

Somewhere along the line, I met a woman who taught me how to meditate. I learned how to meditate with the monks at the Tibetan museum. I started going to Overeaters Anonymous and other things outside of AA to manage my anxiety better. My saving grace was learning how to sit still and connect with my Higher Power, who gave me the strength to deal with everything that was going on. He also gave me the courage and strength to deal with all that was about to happen.

After about a year of meditating regularly, practicing yoga and doing other things outside of AA, I started to remember being sexually abused by my father as a little girl. While I had always remembered my brother sexually abusing me, I had blocked out the memory of my father raping me entirely.

Over the next year-and-a-half, I endured daily flashbacks of memories that were so violent, so bad, that they would literally bring me to my knees. I remembered memories of my father smothering me until I would lay still and, when he was done, leaving it to me to fix the sheets so that my mother wouldn't know he was in my room. I recalled how he came into my room, beat and raped me when I was fifteen. Only one hundred and ten pounds at the time, I blamed myself because I wasn't able to get him off of me. Already an alcoholic, I was drunk and my body responded.

My father would force me to do things and then give me rewards, usually ice cream or a chocolate bar. He would give me extra food at dinner so my brothers and sisters would hate me for being his favorite. He would isolate me from my siblings to have more access to me while my brothers and sisters thought I was getting special attention. He would take me in the car and, while driving through the back streets, tell me that he would leave me on the side of the road if I told anyone. He treated me like a dog, putting the fear of God in me that I would be alone if I ever told.

After he raped me, I told no one about it for twenty-five years. I dissociated, drank, drugged, ate, and spent money. I did all that to cope until I met a therapist skilled in trauma therapy who really saved my life. Looking through the painful memories and feelings about my father and my brother in sobriety was extremely difficult. I learned how to sit and meditate, inviting the memories to come to my awareness so that I could get rid of them.

Of course, I had to deal with all of the feelings that came along with those memories, like accepting the fact that my mother never came to help me, which was extremely difficult. The movie "Precious" depicts her mother saying, "Well, she didn't tell me. She just laid there and took it." That is pretty much what my mother would have said. She had also been sexually abused and would have blamed me. She was so co-dependent with my father that she couldn't live without him or see that there was anything wrong with him. So, I knew as a child that I didn't have a mother I could go to. I knew that telling my mother would have fractured her. The rule in the family of incest is to just keep quiet; keep the family together and we will all be OK.

The beauty in all of this was that I stopped blaming myself for being an alcoholic. I stopped blaming myself for being self-destructive and for being a compulsive overeater. I was finally able to understand where all the self destruction came from and be free. I was able to understand that it wasn't my fault. I also began to understand why I was bipolar, so now when people rush to judgment or make a remark about being bipolar, I can let it go. I realize today that people don't just simply end up in mental hospitals, or in handcuffs and straight-jackets for no reason. I had suppressed so very much trauma underneath my addiction; underneath all of my addictions.

It is almost five years since I remembered the abuse. During that time, I discovered that my daughter had been abused by a nephew who put a knife to her throat and said, "Don't tell anyone." She was able to tell me because I'm here; I'm present; and she knows it. She can feel it. So I brought my daughter to therapy and never wanted to pick up a drink or any food over the situation, which is just a miracle beyond miracles.

Two-and-a-half years ago, in the midst of my own struggle to recover from sexual abuse, my daughter came home from a visit with her father one day and told me that he had molested her. I almost lost my mind, but I didn't because I had to intervene and go through the court system. It took about twenty court dates and a lot of legal stuff with Child Protective Services, the authorities and even the FBI, to ensure my daughter's safety.

Only a few weeks ago, my daughter described the details of how her father had enticed her into the sexual abuse by making it a game. This makes him one of the most dangerous types of predators. While it is still very frightening to deal with my daughter's father, and I have had to move several times in the last few years to hide from him, I passed on the information my daughter gave me to the authorities where he now lives to ensure the safety of others.

My family of origin has been absolutely no support what-soever during all this. In fact, two of my sisters called CPS during this time to have my daughter removed from my custody because they said I must be off my bipolar medication. That is how strongly my sisters didn't want to believe what happened to my daughter. Their eyes are still closed to the familial sexual abuse that occurred. When CPS completed their report, all the allegations my sisters made against me were unfounded and investigators noted that I was one of the best mothers they had ever encountered.

The last couple of years have been really difficult for me but I have not had to go back into addiction to deal with the pain. In spite of all the difficult times, God has always shown me some light, some sense of hope, some kind of peace. He doesn't remove the pain but He helps me to go through it. The Twelve Steps, particularly the Eleventh Step, has helped me trust God and develop a growing relationship with Him which has become the most wonderful and important aspect of my life.

My own sexuality is still very difficult to deal with. I still don't sleep well at night and can't sleep in bed with anyone else because I jump all the time. I always have that third eye looking for an assailant to come into my room. Although it is still very difficult to allow anyone near me, I am working on it. There is not very much I can do except show up, don't pick up, go to my therapy, go to my meetings and let God heal me. I know I will heal in time. I just have to be patient with that and permit God to heal me.

Someday, I trust I will be able to do something immensely positive with my experience, even if it is just helping one other woman. I taught some parenting classes sometime ago, incorporating information about sexual abuse into the class for parents. In one class of ten parents I taught, two families came to me after the class to tell me that they had discovered their own children had been molested. There is a very great need to teach families what to look for and what questions to ask. At some point, I will probably teach more parenting classes in the hope that I can give back as much as I have been given.

I'm very grateful to the former Miss America, Marilyn Van-Derbur, who wrote about her life experience with incest in "Ultimate Betrayals." I commend people like Larry King and Oprah for starting a dialogue about addiction and incest. We have so much further to go but help is truly available for anyone who needs it and there is much hope.

The grief of not having a family has been horrific. I am grateful for all the people God has put in my life and my daughter's life, many of whom are in 12 step programs. While some of these people have become our pseudo-family, I have learned to stay away from anyone who takes the approach that if you don't do it my way, if you don't tally up your columns this way, you can't be in our circle. I was excluded from my biological family, but I am not excluded in program. It is my choice in program who I am friends with and who I merely say "hello" to.

In other words, I can't afford to just walk around thinking that the program is not right for me because of a few individuals. There is plenty of goodness in 12 Step programs. I am very grateful for those programs and all the mental health professionals who have helped me along the way.

For today, I have given up having the big career in order to take care of my most cherished gift, my daughter. Working part-time as an Administrative Nurse is the perfect job for me because I can use my "book-smarts" while having the flexible schedule I need to be a mother to my daughter. I am blessed to be working with wonderful people, including a woman in recovery who is warm, funny and shoots from the hip. She has taught me so very much and she has been such a help to me.

Shopping in thrift stores, doing my own nails and living simply has allowed me to save money. I have a nice apartment and really do have everything I need. About all I could ask for right now would be to have a washer and dryer, but as I am currently planning a surprise trip to Disney for my daughter and me, I guess I'm in pretty good shape financially.

My daughter is a wonderful girl; the very light of my life. Although she is not completely healed from what happened to her, I trust God that she will be in time. She has a good sense of humor, is doing well in school and socializing well, but still feels her pain deeply. She is able to talk about what happened to her only because I am a mother who she can tell anything to. That is only possible because I am sober and abstinent, which means that I don't have the blinders of addiction on me.

I truly know in my heart that my daughter will have a better life than I did because she won't ever be sitting somewhere, crying, "Why didn't my mother protect me?" Ironically, watching my daughter heal helps me heal from my past because I can then find compassion for myself as a little girl. Now that both my parents rest in peace, I am sure they would both be proud that I am breaking the chains of violence and abuse that has gone on for generations on both sides of the family.

While I sometimes think that the cards I have been dealt in life have been very difficult, I am very grateful to God for giving me the courage and strength to deal with them. Although it has taken a lot of help from others as well as time and being patient with myself, I remain very grateful for the life I have today. I know that God has very good plans for me because I am not blocking His gifts with addiction and resentments anymore.

From someone who spent my whole life running, I have what I want most in life today only because I am willing to deal with my feelings. That is really as simple as my recovery gets. I spend time with God and I spend time at meetings. I reach out to other people even if it's just to make a quick phone call to someone I think needs it. Today I look forward to the surprises that God has in store for me.

Life and Career Worth Salvaging

I came from a dysfunctional home. My father was a very heavy drinker, an atheist and a communist. My mother was the daughter of an alcoholic. There were three children, of which I am the oldest. They divorced when I was five.

Mother remarried when I was seven and we were adopted by her second husband who was bipolar with schizoaffective disorder. He abused me for many years. I determined I would never marry.

In order to support myself, I became a nurse. I desperately wanted to be an English teacher or journalist but could not afford college. Writing is one of my joys.

I worked in critical care because I loved the adrenaline rush. I was singled out early in my work history to help develop the hospital's first CCU and I was sent to a university in the Northeast for a four-week course. I was prescribed diet pills and my supervisors loved my performance when I was on them. After setting the unit up and working there for a couple of years, I traveled to another facility for work with open heart surgery.

It was there that I was encouraged by colleagues to "loosen up" and attend "metabolic rounds" at a local pub. I got drunk the very first time and was seldom sober thereafter. Though I never touched alcohol until my late twenties, I can tell you that, for me, it was as if someone threw a match to a can of gasoline. It was soon thereafter that I discovered marijuana. And Valium.

I drank with impunity for many delirious years. I was a hit at the disco clubs; dated many men; even did well at my attempts at a degree in English. Ultimately, during a job for a plastic surgeon, his wife felt I should become a Nurse Anesthetist and I applied and was accepted into school.

My drinking life was consummate at that point, but I went away to school anyway. I believe the only thing that helped me complete the program was the twenty-four hour call that kept me away from the scotch, which was difficult to obtain given the state distributed liquor stores. I dated someone who worked in one of the stores.

When I returned home after graduation, I felt an impending sense of doom. I knew in my soul that I was an alcoholic and that I was helpless against the next drink, yet I could not conceive of life without it.

Still, it was six more years before that horrible afternoon when three CRNAs and one anesthesiologist gathered to perform an intervention on me. I was truly devastated, but admitted to the evaluating psychiatrist that I had a drinking problem. At that time I was consuming the better part of a fifth of scotch or vodka an evening and more on weekends. I would awaken at two or three a.m. and vomit, checking for blood of course; and then I'd drink some more. By ten-thirty a.m. on the days I worked, I would be shaking noticeably.

I was admitted to a psychiatric hospital and began my long journey back to some semblance of mental health. I withdrew; I wept; I couldn't eat; I couldn't even see to read.

At the end of the first week, my psychiatrist placed my chart on the bed during his daily visit and opened it to my lab work. He said, "Most patients would not appreciate this, but I believe you will." Not one of my lab values was normal. My GGT was 1470 (normal 0-40.) My potassium was 2.6. Even my EKG was abnormal and is to this day. That was the advent of acceptance of true powerlessness for me. It was also the beginning of my decision to live and to do it without my old friend alcohol.

My life without alcohol was very difficult at first. There was so much unresolved angst to be dealt with and all in the neuro-psychological condition of early recovery. Still, I trudged a-long with meetings and therapy. I was exhausted at the end of the day and slept remarkably well.

At about six months sober, I decided to just end it all and com-mit suicide with carbon monoxide. I was in the midst of a prolonged withdrawal syndrome and in severe pain. The saving factor was my little dog who would not have survived without me. Instead, though, I called my sponsor and she is responsible for the rest of my journey in recovery because she instructed me to pray. My life of constant self-appraisal, re-sponsibility and spirituality had truly begun.

At about three years in recovery, I became aware through attendance at Caduceus meetings that the nurses were treated differently than physicians in recovery. Nurses were treated like felons instead of like the sick clinicians that they were. So I began my work with the nursing association and Board of Nursing in my state in an effort to develop an alternative to discipline program for nurses. Three of us manned the first state funded pilot program. Ultimately, the Board of Nursing took over the program and it became the very successful pro-gram we have today.

I had also approached the American Association of Nurse Anesthetists in an effort to develop a safe mechanism for re-entry into practice for the CRNA recovering from opiate addiction. My work has centered on the use of the drug naltrexone as an adjunct to re-entry. Although the use of nal-trexone was a novel approach at the time, it is now a widely accepted part of re-entry.

Most methods established to identify, prosecute and bar from the health professions any individual charged with a drug-related offense would have totally missed me and many others with a troubled history, such as mine, on a journey to destruct-ion. I can assure you that the colleagues who did my inter-vention considered me and my practice worth salvaging.

As I approach retirement, my peer assistance work has de-creased. I maintain my relationship with my Board of Nursing and count them among my friends. I continue my friendship with my replacements on the AANA Peer Assistant Advisors Committee. There are so many bright and talented CRNAs and nurses in recovery. It has truly been one of the highlights of my life to get to know them.

I married for the first time at the age of sixty to a man I met in the meeting rooms. He is my soul mate. I have been sober now for twenty-three years and continue to work for, and with, the anesthesiologist who did my intervention. I send those wonderful, caring colleagues who did my intervention a bou-quet of flowers every year on the anniversary of my sobriety. Life is good.

Gratitude For Another Chance

From my earliest memories, I had never felt comfortable inside myself. I had a feeling of uneasiness, as if something was missing; a disquieting feeling that I had been left out or excluded. I was shy, insecure and completely lacking in self-confidence.

In my teens, I discovered alcohol, and I immediately liked the effect it had on me. It smoothed away that shyness so I could be lively; gave me the confidence to have opinions and speak my mind; and most important, I felt connected and forgot about feeling uncomfortable.

I loved the emergency room the moment I set foot in it. In the late 1970s, a few months before my twenty-first birthday, I began working in the ER. I loved the excitement, the importance of what we were doing. It gave me a sense of validity, credibility and power that I never had before. It was with tremendous pride that I said I was an emergency department nurse. Down the road, my title would become emergency trauma nurse but my role as an emergency trauma nurse would later come to be my sole identity.

Life in the ER was a blast. The work was intense and fast, and the nurses and doctors were young and fun. We worked hard, and partied like there was no tomorrow. The parties were outrageous, and while we all drank and used whatever the recreational drug of the moment was, I invariably found that I got drunker or higher than everyone else, or that I was just starting to feel great when everyone else was calling it a night. I was becoming acutely aware that I didn't drink like everyone else, and I was starting to hear remarks about how drunk I got, with embarrassing reports of what I did that I didn't seem to remember.

I was ashamed that I didn't seem able to drink like everyone else, and drinking socially was becoming a problem. I became a liability at parties, weddings and other events. Ultimately, I began declining social invitations, knowing I wouldn't be able to control my drinking and not wanting to embarrass myself once more.

Healthcare took a turn in the early 1980s and changed dramatically, as did the climate at work. Many of the staff members were leaving to work at other facilities, and I, too, moved on and found work in another ER. Many of my co-workers were marrying and settling down. The wild parties were gone; the drugs had long since vanished. Two of the hospitals I worked in closed their doors.

I continued to drink heavily and managed to completely total three cars while drunk in a ten year span. I chalked it up to bad luck, thinking I was the victim of unfortunate circumstances. I vowed, however, never to drink and drive again after the last accident which resulted in a DUI.

Work had always been extremely important to me. I had become an excellent ER nurse and loved my work, but so much had changed. There were far more regulations and rules; less laughter and levity. The camaraderie was gone and I was finding myself increasingly unhappy at work.

By now, I had been working in the ER almost twenty years. Around this time I met the man who would become my husband. He was also an ER nurse. There was the initial phase of early courtship with wining, dining and staying up late drinking; usually later than he wanted to.

One morning, as I suffered through yet another hangover, he said to me, "I'm getting really tired of nursing your hangovers." This raised a mental red flag, but I soon forgot about it. True, on most days off I would be bed-bound for half a day, wash cloth over the forehead, basin on the floor next to the bed in case I couldn't make it to the bathroom to throw up. On the days I wasn't off, I went in to work, undoubtedly legally drunk, feeling like I had an ice pick through my brain. I was starting to drive again after drinking and knew that my drinking was out of control. I became afraid I would lose the relationship because of it, so I had to stop drinking, and I did.

Within several months after I had quit drinking, I became increasingly hypercritical of the performance of my coworkers. I was changing jobs frequently, hoping to find the environment I had worked in during my early years in the ER. I would last at one job about nine months before I'd get fed up and move on.

No one was doing it right anymore. I was intensely frustrated with work and kept trying to make people do it my way. It was either my way or the wrong way. I found myself crying on the way home from work and crying myself to sleep at night. I dreaded going to work, was irritable and miserable, having frequent run-ins with staff, patient's families and even the patients.

I was being called into the manager's office frequently to be "counseled," with the same adjectives being used to describe my behavior: confrontational, antagonistic, hostile and unsympathetic. I felt I was persecuted, misunderstood and unappreciated. I was scared and felt empty inside, but worse, I felt betrayed by the nursing profession.

Before this, I had had premenstrual migraines which were becoming more frequent and didn't seem to have anything to do with being premenstrual anymore. There was a partially used

82

prescription of Vicodin at home from an old injury either my-self or my husband had had and I began taking that.

My headaches went away and I started to feel a little less irritable and frustrated. I used that leftover Vicodin prescript-tion up in about two weeks and then asked a friend of mine, one of the ER docs, to write me a prescription for Vicodin for my migraines. She agreed.

That prescription of thirty pills lasted about three days and I began diverting drugs from work. I was working in the ER of a small community hospital that functioned the old-fashioned way, non-electronically. Re-stocking the narcotic cabinet sim-ply entailed going to the pharmacy with a Xeroxed requisition sheet with what you needed written on it, and your order was filled.

Within the year, I was taking sixty Vicodin a day. One day, one of the pharmacists remarked on the amount of Vicodin our department was using because I was ordering very large amounts of Vicodin to meet my habit. I figured I better order some other medications to detract focus from the Vicodin, so I added thiamine, Prednisone and Demerol to the order.

After I got back to the ER, I realized I couldn't stock the Demerol because the count would be off, so I put it in my purse. When I got home that night, I wasn't sure how to get rid of the Demerol and put it in the back of one of the cabinets in the bathroom, never intending to use it. Although I had used recreational drugs when I was younger, the one thing I never did, and was afraid of doing, was anything injectable. I hated needles.

By now, I was using enormous amounts of Vicodin and I began to become concerned about the amount of Tylenol I was consuming. After looking up the number of grams of Tylenol one could safely consume per day, I switched to Norco. I knew I was addicted at this point and tried to quit several times, but got so sick I couldn't do it. I didn't know what to do because there was no way I was going to tell my straight-laced husband for fear he'd divorce me; so I continued, thinking I'd manage to quit at some point.

Finally, I wasn't able to get enough Vicodin from the pharmacy at work without drawing more attention to myself and the department. So, it occurred to me that I could, in a pinch, write my own prescription, just once, until I could figure out how to get out of this mess. I remember thinking I really needed to think about this problem and do something soon.

I was able to fill the prescription I wrote easily and reasoned that I better back off from the pharmacy at the hospital a bit. So, in the meantime, I just continued to write my own prescriptions. I knew I didn't want a trail, so everything was cash. I memorized fictitious birthdays and addresses for each pharmacy I visited, which became an enormous amount of work. I was prolific, sometimes hitting three or four pharm-acies in a day to hoard the drug if I wasn't scheduled to work.

I had a huge problem on my hands and knew it. Suddenly, it seemed Vicodin addiction was everywhere in the media, on the news, in magazine articles. I still didn't know how to get out of this mess, and felt alone and scared.

One night, I was home with my husband and just about out of Vicodin. There were no excuses to go out and run an "errand" and I remembered the box of Demerol in the bathroom cab-inet. I wrestled with the thought for a little while and decided I had little choice but to use the Demerol. So, I went into the bathroom, took out the bristojects and injected fifty milligrams of Demerol intramuscularly into my rear. I remember getting horribly nauseated and vowed never to use Demerol again, but I kept the rest of the box, "just in case."

It wasn't too long after that when a similar situation arose and I found myself at home again, low on Norco and with no excuse to go out at night. This time after I used the Demerol, I had only a brief wave of nausea. I didn't realize it then but I had launched into a new world of misery beyond anything I could ever imagine.

It didn't take long at all for my tolerance to the Demerol to skyrocket. Demerol was always on my re-stocking order, and soon, as before, in order to move focus away from one drug, I began ordering Dilaudid also. The Vicodin just wasn't holding me anymore, so I continued augmenting my habit with self-prescribed Norco, although I was using Demerol and Dilaudid primarily now.

Inside, I was a mess. I knew I had a huge problem but had no idea what to do about it. I tried to quit numerous times and became unbearably sick. My husband thought I had the flu, a lot. If I didn't use something every two hours, I'd develop intense abdominal cramps, diarrhea, vomiting and chills. My nose and eyes would run.

I became terrified to go to sleep because of the enormous amounts of Demerol and Dilaudid I was using, up to a thousand milligrams of Demerol and forty milligrams of Dilaudid daily. I would awake in the middle of the night with unbearable abdominal pain and barely make it to the bathroom in time. Sleep, once something I found to be so restorative, became my enemy. I would finally get to sleep at four a.m.

Paralyzed with the fear that I'd be found out, or die, I wanted desperately to stop, but didn't know how. I had never encountered a problem that I couldn't somehow resolve and, for the life of me, I couldn't figure out how to stop this addiction. I hoped that, somehow, I would magically wake up in the morning, not wanting to use.

Telling anyone was out of the question because I felt filthy; tainted. I despised myself and had broken not only the tenets of the nursing profession, but my own values and ethics as a nurse. I had become a liar and a thief; a drug addict of the worst kind. I had never met another nurse who had this problem and remember looking in the mirror one day, thinking, "My God, where did you go? What happened to you?" I never felt so trapped or so scared.

I had heard about nursing diversion programs but didn't know anything about them. I thought they were jail for the worst of the worst nurses and I was unwilling to admit that I fit that bill. The realization finally came to me, though, that the only way I would be able to stop would be to get caught.

Things continued to get worse. One afternoon when I was in the car with my husband, I thought he was talking to me and asked him what he had said. Then, I realized it had been me who had been talking. It was like an out-of-body experience and I was terrified.

Two months before I got caught at work, I tripped over a staff member's foot in my haste to get my order into the pharmacy. I fell flat on my face and never extended my arms to catch my fall. I sustained a laceration to my nose, which was sutured. They wanted to order a CT scan of my head at the time but the only thing I could think about was getting to the pharmacy.

Although they wanted to send me home, I insisted on working the rest of my shift; black eyes, sutured nose and all.

Two months later, I went to fill the department order at the pharmacy in the late afternoon. Since the pharmacy worked eight hour shifts and the ER nurses worked twelve, I would fill orders twice a day: once in the morning, and then later in the afternoon, after the pharmacy changed shifts. This time, though, the pharmacist asked me if I hadn't been up there to fill an order that morning and commented that we couldn't possibly be using that much Demerol and Dilaudid. I rather indignantly told her I hadn't been there that morning. When she said, "Just a minute," and disappeared from the window, I knew she was pulling the morning requisition.

I can't begin to describe the panic I felt when the pharmacist wanted me to bring back all of the narcotics I'd obtained that morning. Of course, I wasn't able to do that since I'd already used some of them.

The next two hours were my worst nightmare. I went back to the ER, pulled a medication administration record and frantically began writing fictitious patient names and times on it. It was getting close to shift change and the ER was starting to get really busy. I felt horrible about leaving the other nurse there by herself since it was a two nurse ER, but desperate, I went back to the pharmacy to turn in this fraudulent paperwork. I was still hoping to straighten out this mess that I knew in my heart wasn't going to go away.

The pharmacist told me that she was filing a medication discrepancy and she suggested I contact my supervisor. It was a Sunday and I went home and called my supervisor, who advised me to contact the State Board of Nursing. She said she was obligated to report me to the nursing board and it would be better if I self-reported before she did. So, I contacted the board and was directed to their diversion program. They suggested that I enter a detox program, after which I would be interviewed in order to determine whether I qualified for their diversion program.

I felt a sense of relief that finally this nightmare was over; but it wasn't. Over the next three days, I contacted eight detox and rehab facilities but none had an open bed. By now, I needed an opiate every two hours or I would go into full blown withdrawal, with chills, dry heaves, abdominal cramps and diarrhea. At the time, I had also been working part-time at another job and knew I had enough drugs at home to last me until my next shift there, which was that Friday.

By Friday, however, I still hadn't been able to locate an open bed in any detox or rehab and was running out of drugs. So, after my shift that Friday at the second job, I went to one of the pharmacies that I had frequented many times. It was a pharmacy with a drive-thru, so I dropped off a forged prescription and, as usual, was told to come back in ten minutes.

They had never asked me for identification before, but when I returned to pick up the prescription this time, the clerk behind the counter asked for my driver's license. When I told her I didn't have it with me, she pointed out that I was driving. So I told her I'd be right back and got out of there as fast as I could.

I went to another pharmacy about a mile away that I had also frequented often and went through the same routine, dropping a prescription off at the drive-thru. I was told, "Ten minutes," went to the parking lot of a market across the street, waited the ten minutes and returned to pick up my prescription. It wasn't ready and I was told to return in another ten minutes.

When it still wasn't ready the third time I went back, a red flag went off. Although there seemed to be a lot of activity inside the pharmacy, I nonetheless went back to the parking lot across the street and waited. This time after waiting for ten minutes, I decided to call the pharmacy first and was told the prescription was ready.

As I started out of the parking lot, I saw two police cars coming from different directions with their lights on. I realized I'd been had because as I looped around to get in the direction of home, I saw the flashing lights behind me. That was it. I pulled into a strip mall and got out of the car, immediately blurting out to the officer, "I'm addicted to Vicodin and I'm very sick."

I was taken to jail, where I spent the next five hours. I asked if I would be able to call my husband before they did because I wanted him to hear it from me first. I know he had been suspicious for a long time, but our relationship had been based upon trust. I had never lied to him about anything until my addiction.

The police called him first, though, and told him what happened. As I walked out of the police department after my husband bailed me out, I remember thinking that I was about to lose everything that ever meant anything to me: my husband and my nursing license. My husband had every reason to divorce me. I had become a liar and a thief; endangered our marriage and our livelihood.

Finally, I entered a rehab facility and qualified for the diversion program. I remember being intensely angry and feeling victimized at the time. I was particularly angry at the world of nursing. I felt betrayed. I hated nursing and everything about it. This was one month after I'd been caught at work and arrested and I planned to tell the nursing board to go ahead and take my license; I didn't want it anymore. I believed it was nursing's fault that this had happened to me. I took no responsibility for what had happened and didn't see myself as accountable at all.

This period in my life couldn't have been darker. I'm not sure which was worse: living in the throes of my addiction or wondering what course my life would now take. I was in deep legal trouble, not working and had the extra expense of hiring a criminal attorney. I was placed on probation and endured court proceedings while I wondered if I would be put back in jail.

When I entered the diversion program, I didn't realize that diversion was not something mandated for bad nurses, but a privilege provided to those nurses who qualified for the program. There were criteria for exclusion and the diversion program was stringent, with very rigid compliance requirements. It was a daunting amount of work, to be sure.

I was required to attend a twelve step meeting once a day for a year-and-a-half and was randomly drug tested at least once a month, sometimes more frequently, for the three-and-a-half years I was in diversion. Weekly nurse support group meetings were required, as were monthly self-progress reports. I wasn't allowed to work in the field of nursing for at least six months and once I did start working again, I needed a work-site monitor to fill out monthly reports. I was also evaluated quarterly by a diversion committee to assess my progress.

Somewhere during the first three months of recovery, something shifted inside me. I began to realize no one but myself was to blame. I began to acquire a sense of responsibility and accountability for my actions; that it had been me who got me to where I was now, in recovery and in diversion. I remember realizing, too, that I wasn't addicted anymore; that nightmare was over and I was relieved beyond what words can describe.

The nurse support groups were a type of mirror for me. I saw a lot of victimization and denial. Many of the nurses didn't believe they had a problem with addiction, which only amplified my sense of gratitude that I was sober and had the diversion program to protect me from myself.

I received a huge education in alcoholism as well as addiction, neither of which I knew anything about previously. My husband didn't divorce me; I didn't lose my nursing license; and I didn't end up living destitute on the street - all of the things I thought would happen when I got caught.

I began to understand what sobriety was because I was living it. My life began to take on a new dimension, better than anything I could have planned for myself. For the first time in my life, I felt comfortable with myself and the world. I was truly happy and knew I had undergone a dramatic change. I developed my own identity separate from nursing. I came to realize it wasn't nursing that betrayed me: it was my addiction.

After three-and-a-half years, I completed the diversion program successfully. I will be forever indebted to the nursing board for offering me the opportunity to not only salvage my license, but to salvage my life. Through the very structured program of diversion, I adopted, what I call, "good recovery habits." Now, over seven years later, not a day goes by that I am not immensely grateful to be sober and to have a program of recovery that I am deeply involved in.

I have opted not to re-enter the clinical arena, a decision that is mine alone and not driven by the board. I work today as a registered nurse, and the work I do today is as fulfilling as it once was in the ER. I do not ever want to hold another vial of Demerol or Dilaudid, or another oral opiate, nor have I had the desire to pick up a drink.

I believe strongly that there needs to be more education about addiction in nursing. Despite the safeguards in place now with controlled access systems to narcotics, an addict will find the means to get what they need. To know where to go for help, who to talk to, and that there is a way out, is fundamental to getting this person into recovery sooner. My hope is that nursing schools and facilities will offer mandatory classes on addiction; on what to do if you are addicted.

It is so difficult to convey in words the gratitude I feel to the diversion program for giving me another chance; for allowing me to redeem myself; for allowing me to retain my license. My absolute hope is that the diversion program will remain in place, if not prosper, so that the next addicted nurse scared out of their wits will know where to go. I continue to demonstrate my gratitude through my actions; by taking other women through recovery and helping them to achieve sobriety. In this way, I get to live a fulfilled and enriched life in sobriety.

Greyhound Therapy

I knew I wanted to be a nurse from the age of four. There was never any other profession for me. I never had any other idea or notion of what I wanted to do in life except become a nurse.

I was raised in a very violent, hostile and unpredictable drug addicted family, which meant I started taking care of business from the time I was only four years old. I was really set-up, right then and there, for being a caretaker and trying to get my self-esteem through helping others.

A bright student, I got a lot of kudos and self-esteem through schoolwork. I had strong relationships with my teachers, and later my professors, because I was not really getting a lot of my needs met at home.

My mother was a master's prepared social worker. She was also a prescription drug addict. Actually, my mother was my first connection. From the time I was thirteen, I stole medcines from her medicine cabinet.

My first drink was at the age of eleven, when I stole four cans of Colt 45. I got drunk, blacked out, threw up, passed out and got caught. My drinking history never got any better than that. I was that perfect alcoholic you always hear about, trying to chase that first drink for the rest of my drinking career.

Even though I was an alcoholic from my very first drink, and was exposed to prescription drugs, I never really knew what was wrong with me. By the age of fifteen, I knew I drank and used differently than my friends. I knew at that point something was different and I even knew I was not drinking very successfully.

I never learned how to drink like a lady. I had a very bad

reaction to alcohol, even before I got out of high school. I would become belligerent and maudlin, and all that goes along with being an alcoholic woman.

Whenever I drank, it was to the point of total intoxication. I was a black-out drinker from the start and remembered nothing that happened when I drank. Because I did not want anyone to know I didn't remember what happened each time I drank, I set up a dual life. I was already ashamed at that point. Even that wasn't enough to stop me.

I went directly to nursing school when I graduated from high school. Originally from the west coast, I found a university where you could drink 24/7. This was a perfect set-up for me. I was a very bright student who grasped ideas easily in class. I remember my classmates would get really pissed at me because I could go out, party all night, get drunk, not study much and still get straight A's on my tests.

During my junior year in nursing school, my mother committed suicide from a prescription drug overdose. Knowing full well that she had been setting herself up for that outcome for many, many years, I immediately went back to the west coast and raided her medicine cabinet. I took all the narcotics and sleeping pills that were left and stayed loaded off her medications for the next four months.

Basically, I was on my own at this point; very addicted and very sick. Still getting straight A's in school, there was really no accountability for me at this time. I managed to graduate among the top three in my nursing class and was a full blown addict in addition to the alcoholic I had become before I had graduated from high school.

At the time my mother committed suicide, I was in my

psychiatric rotation at school. It was there that I met a psychiatrist who was more than happy to write me prescriptions. He became another connection for me. I really went straight from my mother's drug cabinet to hooking up with an impaired physician. We would split the prescriptions he wrote for me. So, by the time I graduated from nursing school, I was really hooked on both alcohol and prescription medications.

My first nursing position was on-the-job training in an ICU. My very first patient was an RN who overdosed, which was to become very significant for me. She actually died in that ICU after taking a whole box of a patient's medication. That's when the total nightmare of using narcotics on the job started for me.

I was one of those people who knew exactly what those medications were doing. I didn't come across them by accident. I was a drug addict and I knew exactly how those medications would affect me. Right from the very beginning, I started diverting drugs and my knowledge of pharmaceuticals did not spare me the ravages of this disease.

In the late 1970's, there were no diversion programs available for addicted nurses. The way that the nursing directors and hospital administrators handled diversion in the workplace at that time was by saying, "You have a problem," firing you and giving you "Greyhound therapy." Basically, they told you to get out of town. Then you just went on to the next job, and then the next job.

I did not have trouble getting jobs because I was bright and articulate, but I had trouble keeping jobs because I couldn't stop my drug use. My addiction was so deep at that time that I would swear to God each day that I wasn't going to use. I'd swear each day that I'd stay clean, but by ten o'clock each morning I had to use to quiet down the cravings.

One day, I overdosed on the job, got found out and was sent home. The next thing I knew, the DEA was knocking at my door and I was arrested. I went to jail, absolutely terrified. I really had no idea what to do. I just thought that I was this bad nurse, a horrible person. This was long before the time when Betty Ford brought the awareness of alcoholism out of the gutter and into the White House.

I ended up having ten felony narcotic convictions and I tried desperately to stay clean and sober. I knew nothing about Alcoholics Anonymous, recovery or where to go. I was very depressed, despondent, ostracized and isolated.

Then in 1982, I got a DUI when drunk and in a black out. I remember thinking about my life, wondering what was going on with me and had what I consider to be one of my first spiritual awakenings. A miracle happened. I realized I was an alcoholic and a drug addict. I saw clearly that using alcohol and drugs wasn't my solution anymore. It was my problem. I recognized I wasn't a bad nurse or bad person. I came to realize that trying to make myself "feel better" by medicating myself with drugs and alcohol was actually my problem.

It was at this time that I went to my first AA meeting which actually happened to be a conference of thirty-five hundred alcoholics in recovery. The very first person I met there was a recovering nurse, which was another miracle.

Up to that point, I had never believed, even in my wildest dreams, that there would ever be another person in the world who had done what I had done. My shame, guilt, remorse and inability to share what was going on with me were killing me.

96

I mean, when you're a nurse-addict, you just don't go up to your boss and say, "Hey, guess what? I'm diverting narcotics from the locker."

Very active in the AA program from that point, I got clean and sober. I started working as a consultant to help hospitals raise awareness regarding the issue of impaired nursing in the institutions in my area. This was very important because facilities had such denial at the time. In fact, it was just about this time when the diversion program for nurses was being established in my state.

I started working in the community and did really well for about ten years, until I hurt my back at work while lifting a patient. I had a blown disc and was given pain medication for the injury. After I had back surgery, I continued to use pain medication. So, after ten years in recovery, my addiction was reignited in 1992.

Those next ten years just about killed me. Even though I had all this information and knowledge about sobriety, I did not really know much about the neurobiology of addiction at the time. I just thought I was this wicked-bad person again and I actually stayed strung out for the next ten years. It is really just by the grace of God that I didn't die.

I had this chronic relapsing, over and over for the next ten years; relapsing and getting clean; relapsing and getting clean. Recovery just didn't take hold because I never thoroughly got the idea that I could not drink or use in safety; that I could not drink or use drugs without punishment. It was like I was on a kamikaze death mission for ten years from 1992 to 2002. I was being treated in methadone clinics and had gotten up to a dose of three hundred sixty milligrams of methadone a day, which I was mixing with benzos and all kinds of stuff.

I knew I was dying, just getting sicker and sicker. My life had narrowed to the point where I was really living in the back room of my apartment, just watching cable television 24/7. I never answered my phone and I was so isolated that nobody ever called me anyway.

At this point, I had moved to the east coast with my soon-to-be ex-husband. He couldn't take my addiction, nor could I, so I wound up in a little detox facility in the northeast that could only keep me for a few days. It was there in 2001, just about half dead, that a physician handed me a brochure for another facility which had a specialized track for addicted healthcare professionals. He told me quite candidly, "I don't know what needs to happen for you but do whatever you can to get to this place."

I was on such a high dose of methadone at the time, that it took me about eight months to detox down to about sixty milligrams before I could be admitted there. By the time I got admitted, I was so sick and desperate that I made the decision I'd either do this and get it this time, or I'd kill myself. God knows I had been trying unsuccessfully to kill myself for some time and, although not overtly suicidal, I was taking such vast quantities of different drugs, passively hoping I would never wake up.

Something clicked for me when I landed in detox on July 25th, 2002. I paid attention to what people told me. I realized that I was not bad, but that I was very sick. I am very grateful that I was able to remain in formal treatment there for three solid months.

This began my slow, deliberate recovery, taking one step at a time. I got a job in a health food store because I had gotten turned into the nursing board again when I had shown up on the job really loaded on my own prescription medications. So I didn't have a nursing license anymore. I called my job at the health food store my "get-well job" and it was there that I got into vitamins and nutrition. I stayed clean and sober and got a sponsor and worked the steps.

In 2004, my nursing license, which had been surrendered, was reinstated. I started working in the local addiction treatment center where I had been detoxed so many times I'd lost count. I became an addiction professional in that facility and became very well-versed in the neurobiology of addiction while working there for about five years.

I took this knowledge, along with my education, experience and hope, and went on to become a clinical instructor in a baccalaureate nursing program, teaching psychiatric, mental health and substance abuse to nursing students. Later on, I was recruited to work in a treatment center outside the United States which had an international clientele. My chief assignment while there was to bring higher standards of criteria from the American Society of Addiction Medicine to the local staff.

Being clean and sober since July 2002, my life is completely different today than it once was. I realize what was wrong and clearly know the nature of my malady. One of my goals and missions in life is the desire to share with other addicted clients exactly what is going on in their brain and explain why they do what they do.

My life revolves around sobriety and recovery. I am still an active member in Alcoholics Anonymous. I have a job in my home group where I'm accountable and committed. I show up and do what I say I'm going to do. I carry the message of experience, strength and hope in my own recovery and in my professional life.

It is very clear to me however, that working in the field of addictions is not my recovery program. I think one of the reasons I have been successful in recovery, as well as professionally, is because I have never confused what I do for my professional career versus what I do for my recovery as a sober woman. My recovery program is about being of service and following the 12 Steps of Alcoholics Anonymous. That is not the same as my professional role.

Wherever I am, whether back home in the U.S. or here in another country, I keep a really clear, distinct boundary in AA meetings. I am never in the AA meetings as a nursing or addiction professional. I am there because I, too, suffer from this malady and don't ever want to drink or use again.

All of the issues with the nursing board have been cleared up for many years now. I have been practicing successfully since my license was reinstated in 2004. I have been working with the board in my state and other addicted professionals. I let others know that they do not have to be alone in this terrible nightmare of a disease.

Our profession is getting better at responding to addiction in nurses but does not really allow nurses full freedom to ask for help. There is still a whole lot of stigma out there. Nurses are terrified to say, "I have a drug problem and I'm really, really scared."

Someday I hope that by working and connecting with others that the level of awareness regarding addiction will be raised. I hope that people with addiction will be accepted with the open arms we currently extend to everyone who has any other treatable illness.

My hope is that nurses will not end up dying behind a locked bathroom door in a hospital somewhere. This will always be my motivating force. I love working with the addicted professional, especially nurses, physicians and pharmacists; all the people who have the keys to the kingdom.

Healthcare professionals usually have to get very sick before anybody speaks up about what they see. I think because of the stigma that's attached to addiction, even when quite obvious signals about what somebody is suffering from are there, nobody talks about it; or people wait until the person has a car accident; or people wait until the disease progresses to a point where it can no longer be ignored.

Unfortunately, there is still some professional denial as well as educational denial present, even today. There are still alcoholic students, addicted students, who are going through nursing programs. I know this because there were students I became aware of as a clinical instructor. I would bring information out of the dark corners and put it in the spotlight for them. I'd tell students, "Here's the place to go if you are having difficulties. There are communities out there and connections to be made so you don't need to be alone. Help is available."

It is so important to just keep talking about addiction as an occupational hazard. We have to become more comfortable speaking up about what we see. We must trust our intuition and our observations, our assessment and diagnostic skills. Using our assessment skills is so very important.

I frequently hear nurses say that they knew a colleague was drug-addicted; yet they didn't say anything. Though we understand the shame and the stigma currently associated with addiction, we must begin to talk about it openly and candidly, just like diabetes and heart disease, or any other chronic illness.

We also need nurses in long-term recovery to come out of the shadows and say, "Hey, I have this illness. This is what I did and this is how I got my life back." We must help people become comfortable speaking up and also become comfortable calling it what it is: a treatable illness called addiction.

Because once you do that, you might just save somebody's life. This is not ever about whether a person, a nurse, is good or bad. This is about whether or not a nurse you know is going to die in a bathroom, or somewhere else, of an overdose.

Clean And Sober Nearly A Quarter Century

From an early age, I was taught right from wrong and always tried to do what was right. I grew up in a loving, fundamental Christian home and remember being a bit religious as a child. I was raised by my mother who had to work quite a bit. I had a pretty happy childhood, except for the absence of my father who died when I was very small. It was somewhat painful not having a father around.

My first experience with any type of mood-altering drug was around fourteen when I found some beer my older brother had and drank some. I remember getting somewhat high from it but found out very early-on that alcohol was not something I could tolerate. I had very few experiences with alcohol after that and those that I did have were not very pleasant at all.

When I was approximately sixteen years old, my brother, who was two years older than I, introduced me to marijuana. I remember the first time I smoked marijuana because I thought, "This is it!" It was the best feeling in the world and it made me feel very comfortable and relaxed. I had always had low self-esteem as a child and that went away with marijuana. Whenever I smoked it, I felt relieved from any inner anxiety I had.

From probably the age of sixteen to thirty, I became a daily marijuana smoker. The only days that I did not smoke it were the days I was out of it; and those were always days I spent actively trying to find more of it to smoke.

I guess you could say that I was a "pot head." I thought that I could smoke it and nobody would know about it. I developed a pretty good tolerance to it and could function well at work

103

even with a pretty good buzz. My grades and my ambition did not seem to suffer at all.

In high school, I worked in a hospital as an orderly and decided to go into nursing. I smoked pot all the way through nursing school and was a very good student. Although I did quite well, I do remember one day at a clinical site being asked, "Why are your eyes so red?" This kind of hit me with the thought, "Does anyone know?"

Overall, I felt I was getting away with something that nobody knew about. A few times my mother actually found stuff and would question me about it. She'd try to talk to me, but it didn't really stop me. So, I finished nursing school at twenty-two and started working. I continued to smoke pot and didn't really take too many other drugs. Occasionally, I did take some psychedelic mushrooms, but I didn't really care for the way they made me feel.

I really felt some pride that I did not drink alcohol and felt that smoking pot wasn't hurting anybody. I felt I was a bit better than the common person going around drinking and driving, although I was impaired on multiple occasions under the influence of marijuana when driving.

Around 1977, about two years after I had started working as an RN, I remember taking home some morphine from the hospital, just to see how it would feel. It gave me a pretty good buzz but didn't hit me like marijuana. I didn't really take anything else home from work for awhile but eventually took some Demerol, which I liked a little better than the morphine. Occasionally I would take some medication from the waste leftover because that was easy taking.

I was single, working the night shift, so if I took any Demerol, I would take it when I got home and sleep all day. Of course, my use progressed to where I was taking more, and more, and more, and I was getting paranoid that people were going to find out. Some people were becoming somewhat concerned about my behavior at work, so I left that job before I was ever confronted, thinking that would stop the problem.

So, I started working in a place where there was no access to any drugs. I had no withdrawal and was relieved to be away from drugs. I felt that taking drugs home and using them was all behind me. I thought I'd never do that again and for about the next three years I didn't take any because I had no access. I continued to smoke marijuana daily and never thought that was an issue.

By this time, I was married with one small child and decided to pursue nurse anesthesia. Although I was a good student, it was a very difficult program with some very high achievers in it. It was a struggle just to keep up and I had quite a bit of inner anxiety about that. My level of confidence was a little bit shaky and, in my senior year, I took home some waste anesthesia medication, which was extremely easy to do. That's because in anesthesia, I pretty much decided what and how much medication to give, so no questions were asked unless you went way overboard.

The drug I chose was fentanyl, which I took home at the end of the day and injected intravenously. It was a very smooth high compared to some of the other drugs I'd used. As long as I didn't do a whole lot of it, I could certainly function and nobody suspected anything. I could even talk to my wife after using it and she never said anything because there was no slurred speech or anything like that.

I remember thinking that I was getting back into those same old routines that I had done before and the shame started coming back. I was sure my classmates weren't doing this, although there was quite a bit of drinking and marijuana use by some. As far as I knew, though, nobody else was stealing drugs and shooting them up, so I felt ashamed and realized I was playing with fire.

After graduating from anesthesia school, I got a very good job at one of the clinical sites I had trained at. I tried to keep my use somewhat under control but there was no supervision after graduation, so I really started using. I could pretty much take the drugs whenever I needed to, which was pretty much every day at that point.

Although it sounds strange, I did not take drugs to have on the weekend and never had any physical withdrawal symptoms. I have never quite understood the fact that I had no cravings on weekends. In fact, it was more of a relief to me, like, "Wow. I'm not going to have to load up with drugs today."

When I returned to work Monday, though, the feeling would hit me that I was going to have to get something. It got to the point where I would tell myself on the way to work, "I'm not going to use today." I'd think about my family and even put pictures of my wife and child inside my locker to look at so I could think about what this was doing to them. I even began carrying some 38 caliber bullets with me to work, to remind me that I was going to end up with one of these bullets in me if I kept doing this.

It got to the point where I could not control my use at all and knew that I was under suspicion by several people. It was the early 1980s when I was actually confronted at work. I denied it and the drug test I took was negative because at that time

106

fentanyl did not show up on a regular drug screen. I was just as surprised as the administrator that the screen was negative because I was still smoking marijuana daily.

While I was allowed to continue working, my direct supervisor suggested putting me in areas where there was limited access to narcotics. I agreed to this and, although it was a bit more difficult to get drugs, I was still able to get them. I kept spiraling down and knew that sooner or later I was going to get caught.

One afternoon, I was told to report to administration and I was confronted by several people regarding inaccurate documentation of wastage. They definitely had enough on me to cause a big problem and threatened me with termination. They also gave me the out that they would let it go if I resigned.

In a daze, I remember sitting there, thinking, "This is the end." Although it was so very, very painful to do, I went ahead and resigned. The drive home was horrific, to say the least. I had a gun in my car and really considered pulling off the road to kill myself.

When I got home, I was met by a very happy wife who told me she was pregnant. I remember walking in the door and her coming down the steps, telling me, "We're going to have another baby!" This news wasn't a complete surprise to me. My wife had very recently quit work to be a stay-at-home mom and was very happy, until I had to tell her, "Sit down. I need to tell you something. I don't have a job anymore. I lost my job for taking drugs."

My wife was shocked beyond words. Although she might have had an idea about what I was doing, I think she may have suppressed it because she never confronted me. She certainly was not using drugs and I'd kept my use secret as much as I could.

Lost at home with no job, no career and no idea of what I should do, I stayed around the house for two or three days. I don't remember how I even approached anybody about treatment. I didn't have a clue what addiction was and had no idea of the mechanism of addiction. I had read very little about it in school but what I had read pretty much flew right over my head as far as what taking drugs could do to you. This was something that people just didn't do. They didn't steal drugs from work and shoot them up.

All I thought was that if I just had another chance I wouldn't do it again. I was convinced that I'd learned my lesson. To me, this situation was a one and done. I hoped it was all just a bad dream and swore I'd never do drugs again.

I began making some random phone calls and was able to get in touch with a doctor's Caduceus group, which met once a week. They recommended I go to Alcoholics Anonymous or Narcotics Anonymous meetings in the interim, so I found some NA groups. I had a little bit of pot left and smoked it in the parking lot before going into the NA meeting. The pot was just about gone by now and I knew I was going to have to stop smoking it, at least temporarily, because there certainly wasn't any money to buy anymore.

Sitting in the NA meeting, I wasn't terribly impressed and was glad to leave after an hour. I went to the Caduceus group and told my story to all the doctors and dentists, who were all very confrontational. I was extremely depressed and asked one of the doctors, a psychiatrist, if I needed some antidepressants. He just laughed, and said, "Anybody would be depressed if they went through this. It's a reactional depression and anti-depressants won't help. You have to deal with your issues."

Most of the Caduceus group members had been in extensive, long-term treatment. They said that I needed to go into such a program, but I just couldn't see myself leaving my family to do that. I needed to find work and even went to a convenience store for a job. In looking back, I was so stupid because I just blurted out to the storeowner that I was a nurse anesthetist who had just lost my job because of drugs. I still remember how he looked at me, like he couldn't trust me to work any-where near his cash register.

Since I couldn't even get a job at a convenience store, my wife went back to working full-time and we sold some things in the home, just to get by. I went to work as a day laborer, although there was very little work there.

I got a job collecting money from people who bought tickets for a barbeque. I drove all over the city and used half a tank of gas to collect these telephone solicitations. Of course, everybody dodged me and nobody paid me for the tickets they ordered. At the end of the day, the guy who hired me felt sorry for me and gave me five dollars, so I actually lost money that day.

There was a little treatment center with a six-week outpatient program in the city I lived in that agreed to take me. I paid the outpatient treatment program three thousand dollars, which was a tremendous amount of money back in the 1980s, for five evenings a week, with a little group therapy. In looking back, I essentially paid them that money to take me to AA meetings.

All the doctors at the Caduceus meeting still told me that I

109

needed long-term treatment, but outpatient was my easy way out. Throughout that six-week program, I just wanted to get back to work in anesthesia and was convinced that I'd never, ever use again. I thought all that was in the past and I had learned my lesson.

It was the first time in fifteen years that I hadn't smoked pot and I was experiencing some sleep disturbances and anxiety. Although some of these symptoms may have been due to the horrific circumstances I was facing, I attribute them mostly to withdrawal from marijuana, which is strange because I never experienced withdrawal from narcotics even though shooting up massive amounts.

I talked to a lady at a homecare agency about a job and told her everything that happened. She appreciated my honesty and offered me a position taking care of an AIDs patient. This was back when little was known about AIDs, so most people did not want to work with these patients. I agreed to take care of him, which gave me a lot of time to sit and reflect.

By the time I finished the six-week outpatient program, I was going to a support group for nurses which I got more out of than outpatient. It was mostly nurses who were on probation. This was before there was any type of diversion or alternative to discipline programs anywhere.

The agency liked me because I did my work well, so when the AIDs patient died, I got another homecare case. The second patient was on Dilaudid which I had not been around much and had never taken before. Sitting there at two o'clock one morning, I decided to take some Dilaudid, which gave me immediate relief from my depression and anxiety, followed by the thought, "What have I just done?" Here I had been saying that I could go back to anesthesia and that I was never going to take drugs again, and the first thing I did when left alone with some Dilaudid was shoot up.

I was totally disgusted with myself and could not believe that, after telling myself that I was through with taking drugs, I was taking them again. The self-loathing was just hard to describe and I really hated myself, but I didn't even take it just once. I took it on other occasions, all the while hating myself and taking it again.

There was no way out for me, so I started to consider killing myself. I felt that my family would be better off without me because I had a small life insurance policy. If nobody found out it was actually suicide, my family would get a little bit of money and I would be able to leave my wife and child without the shame that I brought on them.

While I didn't tell anyone at the nurses' group that I was using again or planning to hit a bridge head-on with my little compact car, they must have known what I was thinking because they quickly made some phone calls. One of them actually worked in a psychiatric unit and before I knew it, my wife was there to pick me up and whisk me away to a psych unit.

The first night in the psych unit I spent sleeping on the floor of the padded room because there wasn't a room for me. It was pretty bizarre waking up the next day in a mental hospital which wasn't a drug treatment center by any stretch of the imagination. I was there with people who had mental disorders but I obviously had as much of a mental disorder as any of them had.

I began to think, "Those guys at the Caduceus group were right. I need to go into long-term treatment." So, after having tried to do it my way, which was a total failure, I called one of

111

the Caduceus doctors from the psych unit who made some phone calls for me. He was able to find a place that was long-term, affordable, and open-ended, because they weren't sure how long I'd need to be there.

After discussing my plan for long-term treatment with the psychiatrist on the unit, I remember a psychologist telling me that my chances of overcoming addiction were not very good. That was pretty depressing to hear; yet, at that time, there were probably not many people with my history who went back to working around drugs who stayed sober.

My pregnant wife dropped me off at the center which treated an awful lot of nurses, doctors and dentists and other professionals, as well as the common variety alcoholics and drug addicts. Since I didn't have any physical withdrawal, I was moved pretty rapidly to a halfway house and put into a group apartment with six other men. I stayed there about three-and-a-half months, which was extremely good for me. We talked non-stop recovery, for twenty-four hours a day, seven days a week and I should have gone there in the first place.

After I got discharged, I went to AA meetings every day and sometimes twice a day, just like I'd been told. While I never really embraced AA and NA like a lot of people did, I heard a lot of good things there. I just never really had that connection which a lot of the people in treatment found in the 12 step program. It seemed like they suddenly found a God or Higher Power, a spiritual presence, and developed a relationship with God they never had; whereas I'd had that and gotten away from it. I pretty much already knew I was never going to get clean without the help of God.

Clean for several months now, I started looking for a job. The nursing board hammer hadn't yet come down, so I still had my nursing license and was able to get a job at a drug treatment center that had just opened in my home-town. Although, as a rule, they required at least a year of sobriety to work there, they hired me as an RN for the night shift. I worked there for about seven months. There weren't any drugs for me to give and I was surrounded by people in recovery.

Still dealing with shame and remorse beyond description, I would wear a cap to the grocery store, hoping that people I ran into from work wouldn't see me. I couldn't bear to face them and have them ask, "What happened?" At church, I just kept away from people because I hated them to ask how work was since I was no longer in anesthesia. So the shame and remorse just followed me around.

Since I had been reported to the Board of Nursing by my emp-loyer when I was terminated, I met with a lawyer and called the investigator, admitting I'd been taking drugs and was getting help. The investigator said it would be quite awhile before the nursing board would make a decision in my case and I should just continue on in recovery.

About this time, I called the man who hired me when I got out of anesthesia school. I wasn't looking for him to re-hire me because he had moved away, but I felt I needed to tell him what had happened. When I told him that I had started taking drugs after he left, was terminated and went through treatment, he told me he hated to hear that. He also said that I might be able to find a hospital or anesthesia group willing to give me a second chance, but in his experience people in recovery with access to drugs had a tendency to relapse.

Several days later, he asked if I'd be interested in doing some vacation relief work for him, stressing that this was a one-shot deal only. If I relapsed, he said he would do everything in his power to make sure that I never worked again. He wasn't even sure I'd be able to be credentialed at the hospital and told me if I had any cravings or desires to use to tell him immediately and he would get me out of there. With eleven months in recovery, I jumped at this opportunity and went back to anesthesia work.

Prior to that, I had heard about a new drug called naltrexone, which is an oral opiate antagonist which was extremely expensive at the time, about five dollars for one pill. I discussed taking naltrexone with my addictionologist who thought it was a good idea in my case. Although the guy who hired me had never heard about naltrexone, he agreed to administer it to me at work.

Although there was an initial feeling of dysphoria and headache when starting on the naltrexone, after about twenty-four hours that feeling subsided. I did really well on naltrexone because although I was around drugs that I had used previously, I actually had no desire to take them. I continued with my AA and NA meetings and I had random urine drug screens weekly to show the board that I was clean.

Two weeks after I started working in anesthesia, I finally got the letter from the nursing board. When I went down to talk with them, I basically told them that I'd been clean for eleven months, had just gotten a part-time anesthesia job, was working at a drug treatment center and had started taking naltrexone. I'm not sure they even knew what naltrexone was but they said they would look into it.

When the nursing board got back to me, they said that they were in agreement with what I had done and placed me on three years of probation. They required random drug screens, quarterly reports from my employer and monitored naltrexone participation, documented by my employer. So, I continued working one weekend a month doing nurse anesthesia relief and working nights at the drug treatment center.

After about a year, I was offered a full-time position in nurse anesthesia at another facility, which I jumped at. Again, people there were very nice and the naltrexone was administered to me at work. I stayed there for a year until the place that initially hired me for relief work asked me if I would go full-time. I accepted their offer and have been working there, clean and sober, ever since July 15th of 1986.

Although I really didn't think I was going to use drugs when I went back into anesthesia, I stayed on naltrexone for the entire three years I was on probation, plus a few months. While I felt pretty confident that I'd stay clean and sober, I wasn't one hundred percent certain because in the back of mind I recalled that I hadn't thought I was going to use Dilaudid either, but I did.

Naltrexone took away the option to act on impulse, grab some drugs, run off to the bathroom and get high. For that reason, it was a very good adjunct for me when going back to work because even if I took a boatload of fentanyl, I was not going to get high at all.

I would suggest to anybody in treatment that 12 step programs be given your best shot. Though it's not the only way, it may very well be the easier way because it offers an outline: go to meetings, get a sponsor, read the Big Book. There is no other outline I know of to offer anybody, even though it may not be the only way to get and stay clean and sober.

I once read that AA is not just a tunnel to another meeting but a bridge to another life. To me that tunnel is a way to get on with life as well as to stay sober. Although I never fully embraced AA, going to meetings everyday is a much better alternative than using drugs. If that was the only way I could stay sober, I would do that. But whatever anyone does, it is never easy.

For about eight years now, I haven't gone to AA since I went with a fellow CRNA who got into treatment for alcohol and drug addiction. He was the one who told me about the internet group Anesthetists in Recovery, or AIR, which was starting up at the time. It's a very good group with a lot of networking and help available so I joined it, still use it and occasionally post on it. I do not disagree with AIR being very 12 step-oriented, even though that is not the path that I took after my early years in recovery.

I am very careful not to do or say anything that prevents anyone from following the 12 step advice on AIR, simply because what I did may not work for anyone else. I really consider myself to be one of the lucky ones because the desire to use has been removed from me. Maybe I just got fed up or God removed it, but I do know that something happened to me in long-term treatment that stopped my desire to get high again. I wish I could bottle it up and sell it.

Today, I look back on my drug-use and think, "Did I actually put a tourniquet around my arm and shoot into my vein?" That is so foreign to me today but back then if I'd had the opportunity to lock myself in a room full of drugs, I would've probably shot up until I died.

I don't think anyone can underestimate what time living sober does because time is your ally. Getting time and experience living through trials and tribulations without having to self-medicate with any kind of drug helps you because you learn how to deal with stress without using. Everything hasn't been roses in my life and it won't be in the future; but I've learned how to deal with life without having to self-medicate or numb myself.

Until I got sober, I'm not sure I ever experienced sex without being high. While I wasn't always shooting up, I was always smoking pot and sex is different when you're not high. I had to learn how to perform and that you could have sexual relations, without being high. That was strange at first and it was one of the more difficult things I had to learn in sobriety. I had to learn other little things, too, but I've overcome those as well over time.

I'm pretty confident that I can deal with anything without using, even devastating deaths and failures that life throws at me. When my only brother suddenly died several years ago, it was devastating, but I never thought I needed to drink or get high. I've lived enough of my life now without having to do that and feel confident that I could handle any situation, even if it were my wife or child who died suddenly. Even though an event like that would be utterly devastating, I could handle it without chemicals.

Time is the only thing that tests you for that and I'm hoping and thinking that I have enough time behind me that I'm not going to have to return to taking drugs, ever. Even if I live to the ripe old age of eighty, and do not have to worry about working or getting fired, I don't think I'll have the desire to use.

While getting on my motorcycle for a two or three hundred mile trip is something that helps me clear my head today, I cannot offer that as a way for anybody, even myself, to keep sober. Yet, it is something that helps me reduce stress and relax, and everybody can find things besides drugs that help with stress relief.

I never heard of anyone relapsing who didn't say it was a whole lot worse the second time around. I think once you get a taste of being in recovery, the self-hatred of relapse is so intense because you know what you've thrown away. In looking back to what happened to me the first time, I can blame some of it on ignorance because I had no concept of what addiction or recovery was at the time. With the education and experiences I've had, I am convinced that if I relapsed now, I would not survive.

I'm just not the same person I was at twenty-nine when I stopped using drugs. I'm a fifty-four year old guy, not an old man, but a whole lot older than a thirty year old, and there's been a whole lot of water under that bridge since then. Life has been really good to me and I'm really on the down slope of my career, looking towards retirement. I have no clue why exactly I have remained clean and sober for nearly a quarter of a century now. All I know is that I just don't have a desire to get high anymore. I hope by reading my story someone can be helped and prevented from living through the nightmare that I experienced.

Graced by the Gift of Sobriety

I read an article once that noted when someone has a predisposition to addiction or alcoholism, if they are exposed to substances in their childhood, that exposure flips a switch in their brain and that they can later go on to become a drug addict or alcoholic. I never realized that before I got sober, but I remember when I was eight or nine years old I had abscessed tonsils and I was given codeine.

To this day, even at fifty-three, I still remember that floating euphoria that I felt back then. I believe that I chased that feeling until the day I got sober. That article was a revelation to me. Of course, I didn't start taking drugs when I was nine years old, but I did start smoking pot when I was fourteen. Since my sister was the "bad actor" in the family and I maintained an A average in school, my parents really had their hands full with my sister and didn't worry about me.

I went on to nursing school and partied a lot, like many college kids do. Then, I got my first job at a local hospital. I was probably out of school for about five minutes when I figured out how to pilfer Valium and other drugs which, at the time, weren't locked up. I worked at that job for about one year and figured out how to pilfer drugs pretty quickly.

Moving to the west coast, I got a job in an intensive care unit. I was too afraid to steal any drugs that were locked up but did fill my pockets up with the drugs like Valium which weren't locked up. I continued to drink a lot and took drugs from my job, "therapeutically," or so I thought.

My next job was in an open-heart ICU. That is where I began taking the drugs that were locked up. I'd take two Percocet that were ordered for the patient and give the patient one with a Tylenol. I would take the other Percocet and stick it in my pocket. I'd always go back to the patient and ask, "How is your pain?" Nine times out of ten, the patient would say, "Oh, much better," and I'd say, "Great." But sometimes the patient would say, "You know, those pills didn't work as well as the last ones I got." So I would grudgingly take the pill from my pocket and give it to the patient. I did that the whole time I worked in the open-heart ICU, which was five years.

I am one of those people who just do not like needles. That was probably what saved me. I remember there were two nurses who were caught stealing Demerol when I worked in that open-heart ICU. One day they were there, and the next they weren't. There was no diversion program for nurses back in the early 1980s and there were all these rumors going around about those two nurses. "Did you know so-and-so was caught in the bathroom with the Demerol?" Although the nurses just disappeared, that didn't scare me or stop me because I thought, "Well, they just weren't smart enough. I know how to do it and not get caught."

So, I just went my merry way. At about this time, I started dating a resident and got turned on to more and more drugs. I figured he's a doctor and he knows what's going on. I started on my way to becoming a trash can, smoking pot, smoking hash, eating mushrooms, taking ecstasy, doing cocaine and Quaaludes; basically anything that someone put in front of me. I continued to drink and also got prescriptions for Hycodan, which is a narcotic cough syrup. Ironically, this resident I was dating didn't like me to drink, so I hid my alcohol intake while I was with him.

Bored with my job in the open-heart ICU, I began looking around for another area to work in. I started to investigate nurse anesthesia, applied to a program and was accepted into an anesthesia school in another part of the state.

In 1985, right before I went into the anesthesia program, my sister got sober. I remember being so bummed out when she got sober because I was counting on her to get people who could set me up with some cocaine and other drugs when I moved to her area to attend anesthesia school.

The whole time I was in anesthesia school there were no oral medications to pilfer. Since I did not like needles, I tried to take the fentanyl orally but that didn't work. So, I continued using cocaine and drinking through anesthesia school.

One time, I remember writing a big paper for an anesthesia class, back in the 1980s, before computers. I had this thing called a Smith Corona word processor that was a kind of typewriter with a little monitor attached, which was a precursor to a word processing program. I had just finished an entire paper with a big glass of scotch and my mirror with my cocaine on it beside me on my desk. There was a tape loop to save and, when I pressed the button, something malfunctioned. I lost the whole paper, but it didn't faze me. I just poured another drink, did a few more lines of coke and re-wrote the paper. That's how it was.

When I finished anesthesia school, I got the residents to write prescriptions for me, like Vicodin and Hycodan, which they did because they knew and trusted me. They didn't really know any better and I was a CRNA, so they would write me prescriptions without questioning me.

I was probably working about two years as a nurse anesthetist when I read an article in a journal that talked about buccal and intranasal administration of Sufenta for premedication in infants as well as children. At the time, we had Sufenta at our facility although we don't have it anymore. A light bulb went off in my head and I said, "Oh, I'm going to try that."

So, after medicating a patient with Sufenta, I put the waste in my pocket, went home and did ten or fifteen micrograms. I took it; it worked; and that started my journey and eventual downward spiral into addiction with that one discovery.

Over the next year or so, I would sign out a little more Sufenta for a patient than I needed. I would give the patient what they needed, keep the rest in my pocket, take it home and use it. I knew that my tolerance was going up and up. When I could not get any Sufenta, I would take fentanyl, but I needed much more of it for the same effect. Since Sufenta's potency is about ten times greater, I much preferred the Sufenta.

Starting to use Sufenta sublingually around 1989 or 1990, all of a sudden I realize that I'm using a lot of it and this isn't good. I started getting a little bit scared, mostly for my job. I wasn't scared for my life or my health because I thought I'm a CRNA; I know the drug; I can control it; I'm fine. But I went to my sister, told her what I'd been doing and she took me to a 12 step meeting.

After my first meeting, I remember I stayed clean and sober for four days. I thought this was great because I made it from Monday to Friday. So, on Friday I celebrated by getting loaded. I really hadn't gotten the concept of sobriety and this started my hideous, horrible journey trying to get sober, doing it my way.

My tolerance to Sufenta got higher and higher. To illustrate this, someone my size could be adequately anesthetized for an operation lasting one to two hours with about sixty to seventy micrograms of Sufenta while I was walking around and functioning at work taking two hundred fifty micrograms a day. I was truly physically addicted to Sufenta, at this point using it and whatever else I could get my hands on because you really can get just as addicted doing drugs sublingually as doing them intravenously.

By this time, I had been going to AA for three years and had gotten very involved and active in the program. There was a lot of peer pressure in my home group to stay sober which started me lying because I knew sobriety means that you don't take anything which affects you from the neck up.

I had stopped drinking, using coke and extraneous drugs so no one would know I wasn't sober, but continued to use Sufenta because I was physically addicted. By now, if I stopped using Sufenta, I couldn't function; couldn't work; couldn't think. If I stopped, I got sick. I would have all the physical withdrawal symptoms any IV drug-user would have.

Every day, I became more and more desperate. I did this for three years, working every day. Every single day, I would wake up in the morning, and say, "Today's the day I'm not going to use. Today's the day that I am going to stop." Of course, I didn't stop and I became more and more fearful for my job.

Each nurse anesthetist where I worked had their own narcotic box, with each of us responsible for signing out our own meds. No one was watching what I was doing, or so I thought. In the beginning, I would sign out more than I would use and put the wastage in my pocket. After awhile, I began making up fictitious names of patients. In those days, there was no audit, so I would sign a fictitious name and take all the medication home. Unbeknownst to me, things were beginning to look a little suspicious. A fellow CRNA had told my supervisor to watch me because she suspected something was going on.

Finally, I remember one day I had just had enough. I was sick and tired of trying to do it my way. It was just a nightmare. My whole life was a nightmare; a big lie. My life aside from work had gotten really, really small. I didn't really have many friends and nobody was coming over my house.

So I had a big surrender - I started drinking again. That was my big surrender. I said, "You know what? I can't do it and I might as well drink because drinking makes me happy." So I started drinking again. I feel that surrender was what saved me. It was almost as if God was waiting for me to give up doing it my way. It was only then that I was graced with the gift of sobriety.

By now, I was so tired of it. It was so much work to steal those drugs to tide me over if I had time off or a vacation. If I had some time off from work, I would have to make sure that I had enough of a supply so that I wouldn't get sick and go into withdrawal. I was doing things like sneaking into the hospital on my days off. It was like one of those cartoons where you see somebody sneaking around the corner on their tiptoes, looking to see if the coast is clear. Then, sneaking into the narcotic room and sticking the drugs in my pocket; then, sneaking out of the narcotic room; then, running to my car, hoping nobody would see me.

If somebody did see me in the hallway and asked what I was doing there because I wasn't working, my answer was, "Oh, I just left something in my locker." Nobody ever thought to question me. They had their head in the sand, or maybe I was still performing well enough at work that they didn't suspect anything.

One day, I was just done. I just could not think up one more fictitious patient name and put the same patient's name in two different places, with two different medications noted on the narcotic record. That night, when I went home, I said to myself, "Tomorrow is the day I'm going to get caught."

Sure enough, when I went into work the next day, my supervisor came up to me, pulled me out of the OR and absolutely saved my life. He really liked me and we had a really good relationship. He asked me to explain the narcotic entry I'd made. I could have lied to him, but I shrugged my shoulders and said, "What can I tell you. I'm sorry." He was just as devastated as I was. I didn't know at the time that he had some experience with recovery and he pulled me off the job at that point. I went to the Employee Assistance Program and the Chemical Dependency Recovery Program at my hospital and started my journey in sobriety.

I feel that I was one of the lucky ones for a lot of reasons. First of all, I was not fired. I was highly encouraged to self-report to the nursing board. I actually had to go into the hospital to detox and realized that self-reporting to the board was probably the best thing for me to do.

While I was in that rehab unit, one of the addictionologists pulled me aside and told me that he used to be a cardiac anesthesiologist. His recommendation to me was to never go back to anesthesia because I would never be able to deal with anesthesia again. He said that because he wasn't able to do it. He had relapsed and informed me that the relapse rate was huge for anesthesia providers. He said if I was smart, I would find another area of nursing to go into. I was just devastated and horrified by this information and didn't know what to say.

Needless to say, I didn't take his advice. I felt that it was not the right course for me and I have not had the need to experiment with relapse. I just never had to go back out there. I'm not sure why, but maybe it is because I tried for so long to get clean and sober, my way, on my own, and wanted it so badly, that when I finally was blessed with the gift of sobriety, I grabbed on to it. The minute my boss caught me that day at work, my obsession was lifted. I have never had the need to use drugs again – ever.

I remember walking along the street during my first year of sobriety. I had this irrational fear that a car would hit me; that I would get injured and have to go to the hospital where they would give me narcotics. So I was terrified of just walking down the sidewalk because I was so afraid of taking drugs. I never wanted to go through that detox again or ever be in that situation again. I never wanted to go through all that humiliation; all that pitiful, incomprehensible demoralization again.

Since I was in a very active group in Alcoholics Anonymous before I got sober, as soon as I got out of the hospital, I went back to my home group. I shared at the group level where I had been, what I had done and that I had been lying. I was welcomed back with open arms and given lots of love and support. I think that is so key; to be really, really involved in a 12 step program.

The nursing board wanted me to also go to Narcotics Anonymous meetings, so I went to six AA meetings and one NA meeting a week for my first year. Since I felt much more comfortable in my AA meetings, I dropped the NA meeting and stuck exclusively to AA meetings after that first year.

Other than detox, I never went for inpatient treatment. I only went to intensive outpatient treatment, which worked for me.

I realize that intensive inpatient or residential treatment is now recommended for anesthesia providers, but that was not my story. By the time that I was confronted at work, I had a good foundation in the 12 steps.

I never took naltrexone or any of those medications that they recommend for anesthesia providers. It was never offered to me and never occurred to me, so I didn't do that. My journey was that I worked with the Board of Nursing and was out of work for ten months. They actually said I could go back to work after four months, but I couldn't do any patient care. Of course, I also couldn't handle any drugs. So, there was really nothing for me to do at my job, which I still had, because I had not been fired. I was out on a leave of absence for ten months and returned when I could go back to a patient care area.

When I returned to work, my boss, this angel who rescued me and saved my life, sat down with me and we drew up a job description for me where I would be the CRNA who oversaw the post anesthesia recovery room. It was a patient care setting, but I still was not allowed to handle any medications, not even atropine or epinephrine. The Board of Nursing accepted that.

For four months, I worked in the recovery room. When nurses asked if I could give this or that medication, I said, "No." I did nothing that went against my contract. I did everything the board wanted me to do – the random urine screens, the nurse support groups and mandatory meetings. Everything the diversion board asked me to do, I did and, after four months, they allowed me to go back into the OR.

At first, I was not allowed to handle my own keys, so my boss would dole out my narcotics, case by case. This was fine because I was really grateful to be back there. Eventually, I was back to functioning at my job one hundred percent, administering anesthesia, handling my own keys, and doing whatever I used to do. I still had to send in reports and do the mandatory urine screens and was monitored for a little over four years.

I feel that my participation in my State Board of Nursing's alternative to discipline program played a huge part in the success of my recovery. Left to my own devices, I probably would have returned to work way too early to have been able to avoid relapse. At the time, the restrictions and limitations placed on me seemed harsh, but now, fifteen years later, it is apparent that the alternative program saved my life and my career. I had been trying to do it my way for the preceding three years, with no success. They knew what I needed and made sure I complied. I am thankful I got the opportunity to participate in that program, rather than go through the legal system and possibly lose my license and livelihood forever, not to mention my life.

Since that time fifteen years ago, I have no anonymity at my place of work. There are a lot of people at work now who were not employed there when I got sober, but I am very open about what happened. I have had one CRNA call me up and ask me to take him to a meeting. There was another CRNA who was caught in the call room using propofol and I was able to intervene with him. I was invited to sit on the Physician's Wellbeing Committee at our hospital as the only non-physician member, so I also give service there. I am invited every year to give a talk to the class at my former anesthesia school about my experience.

Why is it that I never had to relapse and there are so many other anesthesia people who relapse? I don't know. It could be that I am so aware of how really blessed I am. It could be that I am very active in my AA group, that I have a sponsor and sponsor others. It could be that I was done when I was confronted at work. It could be I realized I could not do it on my own, so I had that surrender moment where there was no longer any denial.

Maybe other people still think that they can control it, or don't really believe that they are an "addict." Maybe others think that they are just using to medicate themselves for their pain or their sleeplessness. Maybe they haven't hit their emotional bottom yet. A lot of people have not gotten back what I have been so blessed to get back, but maybe they aren't doing what I did, and continue to do - really get deeply involved in the program and work the steps, a day at a time, every day.

My Mom Was "My Rock"

My Mom had been in hospice, dying of cancer. As a nurse, of course, I took care of her, even though there were hospice aides coming in. I would work all night, then come by and care for her a couple hours during the day.

Four months prior to my Mom dying, my sister-in-law died of cancer. I had actually stepped-in to take care of her first, before my Mom. Those two women were the two very closest people to me in my whole life. They were the two people I most identified with and my very best friends.

You see, my Dad and my brother were drinking and drugging themselves with marijuana and alcohol, although my brother ended up using crack. They would both party and were very different from my Mom, my sister-in-law and myself. We were the sane ones and we strengthened each other.

So, when my sister-in-law passed away, I remember going to the funeral with my mother. My Mom knew at that time that she had cancer and she said at the funeral, "I guess I'm next." Of course, I didn't want to hear that.

My Mom and I never discussed her dying. She was sixty-eight years old at the time. She was a wonderful, very hard working woman and I was so angry that I was losing her. She would be lying in the hospital bed in her room, look at me and say, "Well, just how sick am I?" I couldn't bring myself to say, "You're dying." I would just remind her, "Remember, I went with you to chemotherapy today?"

It was important for me to spend the rest of her life with her. I had to be the strong one, because my Dad and my brother just didn't get it. I knew they weren't well. So, I would go to stay with my Mom before I'd go off to work, around eleven at night. I'd turn and position her for the night around nine or ten o'clock and make sure she was as comfortable as possible.

By this time, she was bedridden with a Foley catheter and a nasogastric tube for feedings. I had to do Accu-cheks because of the medications she was on and I would inject her with Epogen. I guess I was trying to keep "Death" away from her. She survived only about four months, which is a pretty quick time during which to lose the woman I viewed as "My Rock."

I couldn't allow myself to fall apart at the time because I had to be strong for the funeral. I had to be sure that things were taken care of because my father and brother were of little to no help at the time. I was so well-conditioned to my Dad and my brother being unreliable back then. They were responsible for picking up the flowers and bringing them to the church. Not surprisingly, they were late.

Everyone arrived before them and kept asking me, "Where's your brother?" "Where's your father?" I just said, "I don't know." I didn't have to go there. I knew what they were doing. They had to get themselves high first, before they could come to the funeral. I remember the very first thing I noticed when I saw them at the funeral was the flush in their face. I knew that they had already been partaking of drugs, alcohol and getting high. I was disgusted and embarrassed, but this was them.

Going to the casket before the actual services began, I remember saying, "Mom, they're at it again." Then I added, "You left me all by myself to do this." Losing my Mom, my Rock, was very traumatic for me.

I didn't cry a whole lot, but I remember being very, very lonely. My Mom had spoiled me. I was forty-something when she died and she had spoiled me. But as much as she spoiled me, it was I who was just not having a life; just working and working, trying to make ends meet. I was trying to get my daughter through college. Being all work and no play made this nurse a dull girl.

Emotionally, though, I guess the bottom started with the car accident. That's when I felt finished, distraught and angry. Having the car accident was the culmination of having worked six nights a week for five whole years when my daughter was in college.

I remember I had worked the night before, gotten my hair done and cashed my check. I was going home to get some sleep and was very exhausted. I realized I was weaving while driving but thought I'd make it home.

In hindsight, I pushed and pushed myself, right into the ground. I fell asleep at the wheel and on impact I actually thought someone hit me. I remember my face shoved right up against the steering wheel. The crash knocked my glasses off. I had tremendous pain in my right wrist. It was then that I realized I had hit a big Yukon. The impact was so great that the driver of the SUV said the back seat in his vehicle cracked. The man's son came up to me and asked if I was OK, but I was just in a daze.

I thought, "Oh my God!" I felt this pain in my chest immediately – not cardiac pain, but pain from the force of the impact. I wasn't sure if my ribs were fractured or not, but knew for sure that my wrist was broken. I remember thinking, regardless of whether my wrist was fractured or not, that I had to get back to work. Although I had that night off, I was determined to go back to work the very next night because I was scheduled to work. How crazy is that?

The emergency department doctor gave me some Toradol, and told me on discharge to take Motrin. Even then I remember thinking to myself, "Why don't you just give me a narcotic? I am going to need a narcotic." They put a temporary cast on my wrist and, when I saw the orthopedist two days later, I still thought I needed some Percocet or Vicodin. So, I got the orthopedist to give me a prescription for thirty Vicodin.

Almost immediately I was taking more than prescribed. You see, prior to the car accident, I'd been in the hospital twice for a stomach ailment. I'd been given Dilaudid intravenously, and later Percocet, and I enjoyed that feeling, that's for sure. So, when I got the prescription for Vicodin after the car accident, I took it more frequently than prescribed.

The supply ran out early and it was hard for me to get back to the doctor because my car was totaled. When my father and his wife came up to visit me from Florida, she was able to get a whole bunch of Vicodin for me. She also shipped it in the mail to me, twice.

I remember at that time being depressed and disgusted. The impact from the accident had left a huge contusion on my right breast. The wrist fracture was very debilitating and I was in so much pain. I tried to take the pain medication only at night. I would get up in the morning, take a pain pill, jump in the shower and then try very hard not to use it throughout the day. Then, at night, I would take two pills.

I was out of work due to my injuries from July to September. By the time I went back to work, I was already addicted. I did not initially start out diverting from work, largely because my daughter had pain medications for her own medical condition which I'd take to get me by.

My cousin also had Vicodin and I remember saying to her, "Oh, let me see the bottle. Let me see what the dose is." I'm ashamed to say that when she left the room to get us both a cup of tea, I took a couple of her pills.

A girlfriend of mine who had dental surgery also had a prescription for Vicodin, which she said was too strong for her. She told me she thought Vicodin was a very powerful drug which made me think I needed to get my hands on some of it. So I did. I lied, said I had a toothache, and got hooked.

It was a full-time job actually trying to figure out how I was going to keep myself supplied. It took a whole lot of energy. When I realized the supply was very limited, I started diverting. I am grateful to be able to say that I never withheld any medication from my patients. Instead, I would sign out doses that weren't actually requested or needed by patients. I worked on a very large unit with quite a few patients who were ordered these medications every six hours.

At first, I wasn't nervous about being discovered because the patients had orders written for these medications, but later on, when I looked at the narcotic sheet and saw that my name was on the sheet more than anyone else's, it made me a little nervous. I remember wondering if anyone was going to get hep to this and think, "How come these people only need their meds on her shift and even twice on her shift?" Some nurses shared with me after I was caught that they had started to suspect I was taking it for my own use. But I was in denial, and I would have denied it if anyone had said anything to me.

The compulsion to use! At times, I would question myself, "Do you think you're addicted to pain medication?" I'd say to myself, "No, I don't have to take this and can stop anytime I want to." But I should back up a little to say that there came a time when I was even signing out doses when I was off-duty. That's pretty much how my diverting was discovered because if I were working a Monday through Friday schedule and had the weekend off, I had to make sure that I had a supply to cover me over the weekend. I'm ashamed to say that I got that supply by diverting.

I was just not able to stop. I would get ready for work many, many nights, and say, "Tonight is the night you are going to show yourself that you do not have to use." The sad truth is that by midnight that same night I'd already taken two Percocet or Vicodin. I had to medicate myself on a nightly basis and now know that physiologically I was impaired. Due to the tolerance I'd developed, though, there was no slurred speech or signs that I was under the influence, so I didn't appear to be someone who was using these drugs.

Of course, I never called-in. In fact, I overworked. When I'd be on vacation and they'd call me up to say, "Can you come in because we're short staffed," I was there. While I was fixing myself financially, I had the added little treat of being able to divert narcotics.

My friends were very, very surprised to learn the truth. Not one of them knew and I'm ashamed to say I hid it well. I isolated. All I did was work. I'd come home, do what I had to do for my daughter and myself, and I would sleep. I would do everything I needed to do: the cooking, shopping, laundry, cleaning, but then I would sleep. If the phone rang, I would not answer it. I did not feel like talking to anyone, no matter how close we were.

This was a very dark period of my life. I have a good understanding now, in hindsight, of how it happened and why it happened. I was very angry that life, my life, was so hard. I really had no family close by and my Rock had passed away seven or eight years prior to this.

By being so very responsible, I was doing what I thought I should be doing, but I was not really taking care of myself because I certainly didn't count back then. To me, prior to coming into recovery, I thought it was selfish, or haughty, to take care of yourself. I didn't even know how to take care of myself. I had to learn at fifty-something that it was OK to take care of myself and learn how to nurture myself. Imagine learning that in your fifties! That's certainly OK; better late than never.

The phone call that I knew would come, ultimately came on a Tuesday. I had waited a very long time for that phone call and I'll never forget that day. I had worked the night before and was called on my day off. My unit coordinator said, "The director wants to see you in her office today." I said, "I can't make it today. I have a doctor's appointment." Of course, it wasn't true, but I was trapped, like a scared cat.

I have never been so frightened in my whole life, but was able to say, "May I ask what this is about?" At first she said, "I don't think I can tell you," but she covered the phone and finally came back on, saying, "The director said to tell you it's related to narcotics."

Well, that just about blew my whole world apart. I remember thinking, "Where am I going to get my next dose from?" That was followed right up by, "Don't worry about the pills! You have to worry about your job; a roof over your head; your car payments. What are you going to say to your daughter? What if your friends find out? What the HELL is going to happen to you and your daughter?" So, about ten minutes later I called back to say I'd be there.

Before I went, I made a phone call to people I thought would know how to flush the narcotics out of my system. I scraped up the money for this horrible medication. After I took it, I couldn't go more than ten minutes without needing to stop along the parkway. It knocked the crap out of me. I had abssolutely no strength at all; absolutely none. I felt like a dried bone, both physically and emotionally.

After going through all that, my employer never drug tested me at the meeting that day. All that torture, and they never tested me. I will never forget walking into the administrative conference room. I've been in that room since for in-services and such. There is this huge conference table and since that meeting I always remember what went on that day.

I met with my unit coordinator first, who took me into the room. I was already sitting at the opposite end of this long table when the director came in. She began to question me and had a folder filled with papers. I don't remember how she actually began, but she said, "You have a problem." Well, I looked right back at her and said something like, "No, it's not me." I did not want to say too much, and remember, at least after the fact, that I was in denial during the whole conversation.

As I was actually telling her, "No, you're wrong. That's not true," the administrator who I knew very well just popped in, sat right down and started questioning me. He asked, "Why did you do this? Was this for your use or somebody else's?" I told him I was having severe abdominal pain and diarrhea, which I had been hospitalized for, but nothing was ever found. I didn't realize that those symptoms were probably withdrawal from narcotics.

They handed me the narcotic sign-out sheet, which was highlighted numerous times with my name. I was told to look at it and admitted it was my signature. I was asked if I remembered signing the meds out and giving them, and I said, "Yes." After that, they basically repeated, again and again, that I had a problem and, finally, I admitted it. I was so, so embarrassed.

They told me that I wouldn't be reported to the state if I would go for help; that I would be taken off the schedule; that they didn't know for how long I would be unable to work. I was also told to report to the Employee Assistance Program the next day, which I did.

Walking out of that meeting, I felt like my whole life was over. I was absolutely devastated. I realized I might be going to jail and have no further relationship with my daughter, for who knows how long. While she was working at the time, we lived together and I was the provider, so what was going to happen to her?

When I get upset, I can't eat or sleep, but I also couldn't sleep that night because there was no pain medication for me to take. My daughter realized this and asked if I wanted some marijuana, so I smoked a joint to go to sleep. I didn't know enough back then to think I was certainly going to be tested for drugs in the future. How stupid is that?

The next day, I met with the EAP person who put me in touch with the coordinator of the nurse peer assistance program in my area, who set up an intake interview. When driving to that intake, I was so very scared that I actually thought about turning around and going home. I didn't know what was going to happen. I felt so very ashamed to admit to anyone what I had done, but I went and information was given to me, including rules to follow.

The intake interview seemed to include pretty much everything that ever happened to me since the day I was born. I was told what was expected of me and it was suggested that I go to 12 step programs. I chose Alcoholics Anonymous and think I only went to one Narcotics Anonymous meeting because I liked the atmosphere at AA better.

I also listened to my brother, who was in recovery at the time. I joined a group and got a temporary sponsor, who didn't work out so well. Although she was a nice woman, I actually seemed to wind-up sponsoring her. A dear friend, who realized what was going on, as he was a sponsor himself, suggested that I get another sponsor and I did just that. Now I have a sponsor who is a wonderful woman, really an angel.

When I went into treatment, I was given a drug test. Oh, boy, did I really feel like a criminal the first time I ever urinated in a cup in front of anyone. It was really hard giving that urine specimen while being observed.

The counselor who worked with addicted nurses interviewed me and when I told her my story, I forgot the marijuana I had smoked that first night without narcotics. So when she called me a week later to tell me that I tested positive for marijuana, I said, "Huh?" Then, I remembered smoking that joint that first night.

While I'd smoked pot when I was younger, I had not smoked

any in quite a while, so when I was asked if I had a habit with marijuana, I had said, "No." Having terrible denial back then, when I did remember that joint my daughter gave me, I said, "My daughter and her boyfriend smoke, so maybe it was a contact high." But the counselor said she had no choice but to increase me from three days of treatment a week to five. Boy, was I angry. I didn't think I needed more intensive treatment. Although I probably entered the health professionals' group a lot sooner than I should have, that was good for me.

One thing I've learned through this journey is that there are no mistakes in life. I think I was able to get the program fairly rapidly because I already had a God of my own understanding. I didn't know much about AA and did the ninety meetings in ninety days that was suggested to me. I think I knew there had to be something to AA and those steps.

Watching others come in as newcomers and seeing weeks or months later how they improved was clear to me even though the first step was kind of difficult for me to grasp. I mean, powerless? Powerless over what? While I knew exactly <u>why</u> I had come into treatment in the first place, that concept of powerlessness was a hard concept for me to get.

I knew there were going to be people in treatment who were much younger than me and I probably had a preconceived notion as to what kind of people might be there. Although I'm not a conceited person, I thought I was "different," but, really, an addict is an addict.

I remember thinking, "I'm old enough to be some of these people's grandmother! What am I doing here?" While I didn't want to be there, I wasn't at all resistant to treatment. I was just really embarrassed. It was really hard to share what I had done in front of total strangers because people hold nurses to a higher standard. A nurse-addict is seen as a slovenly person; not by everyone, but by some. They think, "How could you? You're trained. How could you not know that if you ingest these narcotics that you'll become addicted?"

Actually, there was one young man with a heroin addiction in treatment with me who worked in a pharmacy. He shot me a really harsh look with the remark, "But you are a NURSE. How come you didn't know?" I just thought, "OOPS." All I could say was, "It just happened."

Meeting all the different personalities in treatment was a hard experience for me, but it taught me not to judge. I learned that I'm no better than anyone else and that everyone was attending treatment for the same reason: so we could each get what we needed to move on.

Treatment was where I was finally able to open up and discuss being sexually abused as a young girl. It was only when I went into recovery that I found out that my brother, who is about four years younger than me, knew I had been abused. My brother just brought my being abused up one day while we were at the marina, which startled me. I was so angry with him for even bringing it up that I didn't utter a word. He just said that, sooner or later, I was going to have to address this situation in my past. In my mind, though, I was wondering, "What makes him think that I was abused?"

The abuse happened forty or forty-five years ago and I never let it well up in my mind. I would never let it surface and had buried it so very deep. In intensive outpatient treatment, we always spoke about nurturing the hurt child. At fifty-seven years of age, that was ridiculous to me. I mean, I thought that I've "been there, done that," and moved on. So, I just thought that situation had happened to me along the way, but I was certainly not going back there to address that now.

My counselor was aware of the sexual abuse. She would try to bring it up and I would shut her right back down. Every day, we used to read these inspirational books and, sure enough, each and every reading seemed to pertain to me and my situation. The counselor would just tell me to find that hurt child and take care of her.

I certainly had no idea how to go about doing that. While I was in outpatient and doing well, I knew there was an area I wasn't addressing. It was the sexual abuse. Being in the AA fellowship and reading from inspirational books helped. So when the medications were out of my system and I was beginning to heal, I really wanted to get rid of all the dirt; everything and anything that made me feel dirty. I looked forward to being totally clean: my heart clean, my soul clean, and my mind clean.

So, one day the counselor just decided that would be the day. As always, the readings were right-on. Everyone in the group knew there was an issue I held onto and I was finally ready to let it go. I shook; I cried. I wanted to let it go because I knew it was one of the most painful issues I had. While it was difficult for me to understand at first how I fell into addiction, I knew a lot of painful things were stuffed inside and I wanted to be whole.

Although I could say that I was a good person, it's not about being good. It's about doing the right thing. To know that I wasn't alone all that time, that I gave up on God, but He didn't give up on me. So, once I got rid of that stuff, I felt I was able to share anything and everything, even the sexual abuse, at my home group.

Some people say that you don't share such personal things in the AA group. Instead, you share things like that with your sponsor. Although my home group is a fairly large group, mostly men, I felt close enough and comfortable enough with my group to be able to tell that story. I came to find out that my brother, who was also a member of my group, was also sexually abused as a child. I was shocked because I never knew that. He had come out about it in the home group, too, but had never shared it with me. I don't know who his abuser was, but I don't think it was the same person who abused me.

Although my mother thought she was holding us very close, when it's family members, they have access to you. They're trusted. So, while you may think you are protecting your child, terrible things could be happening. And terrible things did happen to my brother and me.

Drug treatment was very cathartic for me and I became looked up to by other women in the group. They knew that I had to surrender my license and they understood what I needed to do to even attempt to regain my license. So, when I finally got my license back, everyone in treatment was so happy. It had been very hurtful surrendering my license.

I've heard other nurses say that when you describe yourself, the very first thing that comes to mind is: "I'm a nurse." Even though I knew it was difficult, I always wanted to be a nurse as a little girl. I remember taking tenth grade English Regents and crying when I failed the midterm. When the teacher asked, "Why are you crying?" I told her I needed to pass that Regents exam to become a nurse. I'll never forget her saying, "Well, you're not nursing material." I was fifteen years old at the time and ignorant, though I now understand where she may have been coming from.

143

I'm very proud to be a nurse. I felt that I had the heart to be a good nurse, because I really do love people and it feels good to give of myself. Being a nurse for thirty-six years now, I can tell you that I love nursing as much now as I did in the very beginning. So, for me, to give up my license was like giving up my life.

When I surrendered my license over the phone, even though it wasn't done face-to-face, I was very nervous. It was a very hurtful thing for me to actually fold my license and put it in an envelope to mail it to the state. I felt like I was giving my whole life to somebody else. Even though I knew that I would get my license back, in time, if I fulfilled the requirements set for me, it was really painful. Of course, I cried.

Out of work, with no money coming in, I had to go to different church programs to get food for my daughter and myself. There were nights we would just eat Oreo cookies with coffee, or milk. I really didn't know where my next meal was coming from. While out of work, I applied for social services and even tried to collect disability, but I was denied because I was a "drug addict." When I appealed the denial, a female judge just looked at me, as if to say, "Get the hell out of my court room, you piece of crap."

Housing was a huge issue because I was in a very expensive apartment at the time. The rent was steep and I had no idea how I was going to pay it, along with my car payment, utility bills, and gas to get to and from my required outpatient treatment, AA meetings and nurses' support group meetings.

Through all this, though, my faith was built and strengthened. More than any other time in my life, my faith was strong. While a lot of my character defects were fear and anxiety, a miraculous thing happened: I was able to let go and let God, and He absolutely took care of me. While there were many times that I was hungry, I was not starving.

When I went back to work after working nights for twenty-two years, one of the initial restrictions I had, like many other nurses, was that I wasn't allowed to work nights. The only day job available for me was two days a week. The employee health nurse, who knew my situation and how I was suffering, got me a third day to work each week to help me financially.

When my health benefits were about to expire because a full-time day position wasn't available, I requested the night restriction be lifted to retain my benefits. I couldn't afford not to have health insurance because I have a cardiac condition and a kidney situation that require regular doctor's care. So I actually worked a little over a month on days and then went back to working full-time on nights. I missed working nights and my patients and couldn't wait to go back.

Returning was very uncomfortable because there were lots of rumors as to why I was out. Some people had said I was fired, so when I walked into the building, they looked at me as if they were seeing a ghost. Someone even came up to me and said, "What are you doing here? You were fired!" All I could think to reply was, "I wasn't fired. I was out sick," which was certainly true.

My friends were very supportive and kind. I was able to talk to each one of them, one by one. When I felt strong enough, it just came out. I had to tell them the truth because they were defending me to our coworkers. I don't know to this day what my friends heard or were told, but I did admit to them that I became addicted to narcotics and diverted medications. I was not happy to tell them that, but all of them told me that they loved me anyway, which was wonderful.

I remember praying before I got out of my car to go into the building that first day back. I told myself "If God is for me, who dare be against me?" It helped me get through so many tough times, especially going back to work, because there were some people who did look at me like I was a piece of crap. It was really hard because I had worked there for twenty-two years when I was finally confronted. I had been the "go-to nurse," mostly for my own shift, but others also looked up to me because I was the "old timer."

Certainly I was knocked down from that pedestal I'd been on and, in some people's eyes, I should have been. I had been very confident and verbal, advocating for my patients, before being confronted. I remember being very angry with people at work who weren't doing their job. I had begun to feel that nobody could do things better than me. I see that now and I have toned that down.

I felt responsible for getting things done. We had patients who were sick and some staff would not pay attention to their symptoms, so I would be the one calling the doctor at one or two o'clock in the morning if they spiked temps to get orders. It just seemed to be laziness and a lack of caring to me. I remember being a patient advocate, but it was much more than that, as if it were my grandmother lying in that bed. I'm sure the addiction played a part in my attitude and, although I wasn't nasty, I was angry and made snide remarks, which isn't like me.

There was one particular nurse who gave me an absolutely excellent report my first night back to work. I like details and she gave me a very thorough report. About two weeks after I returned to work, this same nurse, who would never even volunteer to give a dose of antibiotics for me before, tried to hand me two Percocet in a plastic bag. Like most nurses initially returning to work with restrictions, I was not allowed to handle any narcotics at all. What she was doing got me very nervous, especially when she said, "Here, do you want these?"

This was the very first time I had seen a Percocet since I went into recovery. I had such an aversion to pills at the time that it wasn't tempting because I absolutely did not want to be near it. I wanted nothing to deter my progress in recovery because I'm very serious about my recovery and work hard at it.

I remember drug addiction as swallowing so many pills at one time. I don't know whether it's because I wanted to get them all in to get the effect or what. Thinking about it now, I can say it was a very sensual feeling, swallowing. I guess because I knew what was to come. While I do take medications, as prescribed, to maintain my health, that's a different swallow. The pain medication I took was a very thick swallow.

So, when this nurse offered me the bag with the two Percocet, I just felt so uncomfortable. I don't even understand her actions to this day. She knew that she was putting me in harm's way. So I began to feel I couldn't trust her. I had to make my supervisor aware that this nurse was playing with me, so I reported her, and thank God the Director of Nursing believed me and had faith in me.

If I am tempted handing out narcotics, I use HALT – don't get too hungry, angry, lonely, tired. I focus on the importance of myself, my life and my career. My life is the best it's ever been and I have a strong foundation in God. I do what I need to do to nurture myself today and I make sure that I'm safe.

I think about using at times more than having any real urge to use. A dear friend who has been sober a long time told me once that, "The thought never goes away." When I first heard him say that, I thought, "What the hell is he talking about?" I did <u>not</u> want to hear that. I didn't want to hear that maybe for the rest of my life those thoughts are going to come up. I mean, who wants to wrestle with demons like that? But it's true, and remembering what he said helped me be a lot less anxious about those thoughts. Just because I think about it, does not ever mean that I have to <u>act</u> on it.

There have been times I have thought, "I can take this pill," but the important thing is that I would know and God would know. I am just one pill away from becoming addicted again and I know if I ever pick-up, I'll pick-up from where I left off, which is frightening to me.

Once I was at the medication cart getting a Percocet for a patient and I had the thought, "I'm tired of struggling. Two pain pills would help me forget and take me away for awhile from this pain and suffering." Diversion crossed my mind and I immediately stopped what I was doing, stepped out of the medication room and just sat down.

God was the first thing on my mind and HALT came next. I thought it through: "You have a good relationship with a man in recovery, who has encouraged you and he has given you information to strengthen you. You are happy. This is a temporary situation. It's not worth it to pick-up. You've been in recovery this long and you <u>can</u> keep going in recovery." For awhile, I thought maybe I needed to go home and sleep, or say I'm sick and get away from the cart. If push came to shove, I would do that to protect myself.

Knowing my triggers helps a lot. I've found that dealing with my daughter's situation is a trigger, so I use HALT to check myself – hungry, angry, lonely, and tired. I was probably all four of them this past Saturday night because I want my daughter to have a better life and she just doesn't see it as I see it. So we've been at odds.

Some nurses think I'm crazy to get narcotic access back. For me, it was just part of being a nurse, performing all my duties. It's not because I want to get near narcotics because I have no reservations about picking-up.

Some people wonder whether having access to narcotics is playing with fire. I have to say that it is if you are not working a good program. If you have any doubts, certainly you should not have any contact with narcotics.

In recovery, I learned about my character defects and wanted to figure out how it happened. Not to blame anyone, but to understand the culmination of factors. I know fear and anxiety were embedded in me, cemented in me, at a very early age, though I hid it well.

I grew up in a house that belonged to my grandmother. My Mom, Dad, brother and I lived there and at any given time my mother's sisters would come to visit. When my aunt's husband was beating her, she'd sometimes come to the house with her face all brutalized. So I had this fear inside that her husband would come over to my grandmother's and beat her up.

My mother was also the victim of domestic violence by my father, which created this push-pull feeling in me of loving my father and hating him, all at the same time. Watching your mother get beat, you try to intervene as you grow older, and then you get beat up yourself.

I knew everyone's life wasn't like mine and I guess there was a huge shame about it. I always felt that I needed to withdraw because I couldn't have friends over. I mean, what if someone comes in drunk and gets violent?

Knowing the dysfunction that my brother and I lived through growing up, I still felt I had stayed "safe." I didn't think I was better than, but maybe stronger than that upbringing; maybe a little wiser than that. Looking back now, though, knowing what I know, there's no way in hell I could have escaped from the dysfunction of my father abusing alcohol, or the people coming into our home who abused drugs, and the sexual abuse and domestic violence that occurred.

One of the most important things for me to stay safe now is to recognize my need for rest. It's hard for me to concentrate when I'm tired. My vision, my recollection, is different when I'm tired, so my ability to stay focused is difficult during those times. Staying vigilant with the program is so important and I've been taught that no man, woman or child gets in the way of my sobriety, and it's true.

I don't remember having any formal information about nurses becoming addicted in nursing school. Avoiding back injuries, proper lifting techniques, things like that were taught. But I don't remember anything about addiction in the nursing profession being discussed. In fact, it's a taboo; it's just not discussed, or at least it wasn't back when I went to school thirty-seven years ago.

Many years ago while I was working for a hospital, I knew some physicians who were addicted, but I had no training about how to handle that situation. I am sure education would have been important back then and should be stressed today, even though it wasn't when I went to school. Certainly nurses do tend to get very lax in signing out narcotics. It shouldn't be that way, but it is.

There is still a stigma against healthcare professionals who become addicted. It's amazing to me that we all know that addiction does happen: yet, when it happens to our colleagues, some nurses want to become judgmental. Education for nurses as a requirement for licensure may perhaps help reduce some of the stigma, so people would say, "This is a disease that, like other diseases, happens to many good people; good people who are well-respected and very well educated." After all, it does happen and we need to recognize that.

Every day, I read from "Daily Reflections," which gives me peace, joy and serenity. That word "powerless" is monumental in my life today because I really am powerless over people, places and things. Staying focused, staying centered, remembering who I am, especially my limitations, and that there's a God I can depend on, on a daily basis, is so important. It very much helps me to maintain my sobriety.

I really don't live well in the past. I work hard. I struggle financially like many people do these days, but I'm happy. It's not about material possessions. I have a companion in my life and we have a lot in common to share. I have my daughter in my life and pray that one day our relationship will get back to where it once was. But my life really is "life on life's terms." And who ever said life was going to be easy?

They Were Right In Treatment

I was born in a little town in a rural country in South America and came to the United States at the age of sixteen. When we arrived in this country, I was enrolled in school, unable to speak a word of English. That was a very scary time for me.

My classmates were merciless and made a lot of fun of me. It was a real culture shock. Growing up in a different country, with a different culture, and a different language, I felt isolated from my peers. I was made to feel that I didn't belong. So, I decided that I was going to learn the English language. I was going to graduate from school and be a role model for other immigrants.

One of the most important decisions I made in my life was to dedicate my first whole summer in the U.S. to watching Sesame Street. That's how I learned to speak English. I also took classes with my sister to improve our English, so that by the time I started school again in the fall, I was ready to speak English fluently, and survive.

In spite of my desire and wanting to learn, in my own mind I felt I was a misfit when I was sixteen. I wanted others to like me in order to fit in. I remember I would occasionally drink alcohol when I was a teenager to kill the pain, but I wasn't an addict then. I used to drink a little bit, but it never bothered me. I would drink and then not touch the stuff for awhile. As I look back now, I realize I probably had post-traumatic stress disorder, which led to a lot of the personal difficulties I would face later on.

In 1981, I became an LPN. I loved working as a nurse and, after two years, I went into the RN program because I wanted to do more than bedside care. I wanted to have more autonomy and three years later, I graduated with an associate's degree in nursing.

I moved to another state in 1988 and began working in an intensive care unit. I don't know why, but I started to have panic attacks at that time. The doctor put me on Xanax and it worked for the panic attacks, but I got severely addicted to it. I couldn't go around without a Xanax and had to take three a day. It was then, I think, that I crossed an invisible, imaginary line into addiction.

After working in intensive care for six months, I went to work in another hospital's ICU. That's when it happened. I started diverting. I'm not sure why I started, but when I look back I remember what relief I felt when my patients would experience pain relief after I medicated them. I don't remember if it was physical or emotional pain that I had, but I started medicating myself. I could work better and had more energy. And I could not stop using!

So one day, out of nowhere, I decided to try intravenous Demerol. That was it. I got addicted to Demerol and I began using a lot of it, as well as morphine. I used it for about six months and then turned myself in. I needed help because I was desperate. Even though I was high, I could still function as a nurse, but one day I started hallucinating. That scared me, so I decided to get help.

I talked to my supervisor and they sent me to treatment for twenty-eight days in the same hospital I worked in. I came back to work under a two-year contract and was on naltrexone. I did not have the narcotic keys, so the other nurses I worked with would give the medications for me while I did other nursing tasks. My workplace supported me in my recovery.

In treatment, I learned about addiction and was told to go to Alcoholics Anonymous or Narcotics Anonymous meetings and get a sponsor. Of course, right after I got out of treatment I thought that was crazy. I wasn't going to have a sponsor or go to meetings. I didn't need that. So I never worked a program of recovery or hung around people in recovery because, in my mind, I thought that was BS.

For three years, I stayed clean but right after I completed my two-year contract, I stopped taking the naltrexone. I have no idea why I did that because while taking the medicine I could not use any drugs since it would cause a bad reaction.

After I stopped taking naltrexone and got the narcotic keys back, it was like I forgot all that had happened. I relapsed. I didn't see the consequences; I just did it. I started using more and more.

Back then there was no PIXYS. We just had the narcotic box and would pull out the medications we needed. In the ICU there were so many drugs just flying all over the place, in the patients' rooms and everywhere. So I would go into the patients' rooms to gather up Morphine, or Demerol. Even if the needles were dirty, I would still use them, never having the possible consequences of getting HIV or another disease in my mind. I am thankful today I don't have any diseases due to that.

When my employer came to me, I admitted I relapsed and went to inpatient treatment again. This time, I started going to meetings because I knew they were right; I was going to relapse if I didn't work the program of recovery. I figured I needed to go to meetings, have a sponsor and do things for other addicts in order to keep myself from using drugs.

My employer decided to take me out of ICU when I returned to work after my relapse. They put me on a floor in an LPN position, which I didn't like. It was a big stab, like a big knife through my heart, because I was an RN. My ego was hurt.

This was all happening while I was going to school to get my bachelor's degree, which I received in 1998. Through the school, I was able to get a job as a community health nurse because I'm bilingual. Deciding not to take the LPN position offered by the hospital, I resigned. In my mind, I thought I would never, ever work in an ICU or any area where drugs are available – I just can't.

So, I went to the community health setting, thinking, "Good. From now on, I don't have to worry about giving drugs to anybody. I'm just going to do home visits to the patients." I thought I would be fine. Even though I didn't think I'd have any problems, my disease followed me.

When I quit working at the hospital, I was reported to the State Board of Nursing because that's the law in my state when a nurse is under contract. So I went to the Director of Nursing at the community health center, told her that I was a nurse who had used drugs and was now in recovery. I asked if she would hire me with the order of probation on my shoulders and she agreed.

For the next six years, I worked there and stayed clean. I had a sponsor who I talked to regularly. I went to meetings and I volunteered to do service. I stayed clean for six years doing that. Then, one day, I turned around and stopped going to meetings, stopped talking to my sponsor and started isolating. I didn't want to talk to anybody, and boom! I relapsed.

I had met a homeless person with sickle cell anemia at the

homeless shelter where I was sent to work. I used to give him his medicine and he had big bottles of oxycodone, Vicodin and MS Contin. I remember just looking at those bottles, thinking, "Oh my God. I could take just two pills and nobody would know."

But I didn't do that. Instead, I asked him if he would sell me some of his medication. He started selling me all his drugs every month for six hundred dollars. He could pay his rent, phone bill, light bill, and I had all the goodies. I didn't think about the consequences that came with it.

One day, when I came back to work, I was asked for a urine drug screen because they thought I was using drugs. Of course, the drug screen came back positive for all kinds of things. I did not think people would notice that I was using drugs. I had become a full blown addict, just totally out of control.

At that time I was asked to leave the community health center and was reported to the Board of Nursing for the second time. I got probation again, but was able to get a job at a counseling center for addicts through a friend who knew my story. Even though the pay wasn't great, I wanted to work and keep up my skills. So I started working as a detox nurse at the counseling center and learned a lot more about addiction.

I worked there for about two years until my father died and my son got really sick. Around this time, I was given some OxyContin by someone at the center. Once again, someone noticed I was acting weird, so I was taken to the office and given a urine drug screen. I wasn't fired from the counseling center because I was honest with them and told them the truth about my relapse. Ultimately, I decided to leave that position though because I couldn't fully commit to the job while my son was so sick.

When I reported the relapse to the State Board of Nursing, they added another year to my probation. Today, if anyone checks my license with the board, they see that I have three probations in a row, for a total of seven years, which has been devastating to me because nobody wants to hire me.

After this relapse, I went to outpatient treatment and I really got it this time. I stay clean and sober because I work with other addicts. I work the 12 step program of recovery, have a sponsor and go to meetings. I am committed to meetings and have a home group. That's what kept me sober before for six years and that's what has kept me sober for the last three years.

Looking back, I wonder if my addiction has anything to do with what happened when I first came to this country. But I've learned through treatment and all that I have gone through that I have a deadly disease which has no cure. My disease can be arrested. Recovery is possible if I stay clean without the use of chemicals and work a twelve step program. That's what I do now.

I am doing much better with my recovery, taking my disease very seriously this time. I am sick and tired of being sick and tired; of going through all this pain. The consequences are pain and despair that almost destroys your soul. I had to come out of that pity-pot feeling that I am a "bad person." I am not a bad person, or a bad nurse. I just have the disease of addiction.

Someday I want to get a job as a nurse, but if that doesn't happen, I'll accept that, too. I want to get a master's degree in nursing education. I'm not sure I will be admitted to a master's program, even though I have completed all my probation requirements with the nursing board. I want to do that though because I feel new nurses are not prepared for what could happen to them. If you talk to any nurse, warn them of what can happen, that they can become addicted, they say, "How can that happen?" Yet it can, and does, happen and they just don't understand it can happen to them.

The statistic I read is that one in seven nurses develops some type of chemical dependency. There are a lot of us nurses suffering out there and we need to have more nursing curriculum, instructing students about drug addiction among healthcare professionals. I want to teach and do research in that area because I feel my life experiences qualify me to educate student nurses about the risk of addiction and impairment within nursing.

I have my dark moments but I chair a meeting for nurses in recovery every Tuesday which is good. We talk about all our feelings freely and give each other hope. We encourage one another to go to meetings and have a sponsor, so we can all recover. I also go to a meeting every Friday night. That is what is keeping me sober now – being with other addicts and helping other addicts.

They were right in treatment. In order to stay clean and sober, you must do the work. You must work a 12 Step program; you must have a sponsor; and you MUST go to meetings. I absolutely believe that.

I See Things Differently Now

At thirteen I had my first drink and my first blackout. My second drink was at fourteen and that was my second blackout. My third drink, which I could really say was my third drunk, was at fifteen, when I had my third blackout. I guess you can see a pattern here.

I have an identical twin sister and the whole time we were growing up, I was being compared to her or she was being compared to me. We were never individuals. We were always lumped together as "the twins."

When we were nine years-old, we moved. I really hated the new school. Even though we tried to be cool, we never fit in. Nothing seemed to work until my sister and I discovered drugs and alcohol. That was it! We had arrived!

We didn't get loaded that often, but when we moved out of the house at eighteen, things really escalated. For some reason, my sister didn't become an addict or alcoholic, even though she was probably headed that way, but I really took off.

During nursing school, I was working in a head shop, which is a place that sells drug-related paraphernalia. So I was doing clinical during the day and in the afternoon I was working in the head shop. By this time I was a daily pot smoker and was drinking alcohol pretty heavily.

Then I started working in a pharmacy which was where I began diverting medication. I did a lot of experimenting and tried everything, even antidepressants, because I wanted something to make me feel better. This went on for quite some time. I just fell in love with opiates, which became my drug of choice.

When I was nineteen, I started working as an LPN. At this point, I had all the knowledge from the pharmacy and knew what drugs should be controlled. I would read all the package inserts and think, "People like me are going to abuse this stuff." And I did.

I started abusing things that were not controlled and were not accounted for, like Nubain, Stadol and Fioricet. I took all of the drugs that should have been controlled. For years, I took Fioricet, only crossing the line into taking something inject-able when I couldn't get my Fioricet. I don't know how I never got caught.

After I became an RN and got my BSN, I moved on to a different hospital. I decided I was going to face my greatest fear and work in the emergency room. At the new hospital, I discovered everything was locked up, even the Toradol. By this time, I knew I really had a problem, but there was nothing I could do about it.

So I started taking the waste. We all know the rest of the story because eventually the waste was not enough. That's when I started pulling out drugs from everybody in the PIXYS. That went on for six months. Meanwhile, I had already been fired from another hospital for diverting. I had lasted there for only a week or two, but the new hospital is really where I crashed and burned.

The intervention they did on me was like those I still hear about all the time. They took me into the office and confronted me. My tolerance was so high that they thought I was taking the drugs for a sick family member or that I was trafficking drugs. I knew I was really sick because I was taking all the drugs for myself and wasn't sharing them with

160

anybody. I denied what I was doing when confronted and I kept denying it because I was scared out of my mind.

The hospital let me go and it was the narcotics officer who wound up arresting me and getting me into treatment. It was not the hospital, and not the nurses, but the detective who was the angel who made my life really, really unmanageable. So, I was forced to go into treatment and got enrolled in the nurse monitoring program in my state.

Even after I got arrested, I was in so much denial that I actually went to the bar to celebrate getting out of jail. While the detective investigated me, I got a job in a pharmacy. I worked there for about a week before I was fired for diverting.

It takes what it takes because after being fired from two hospitals and a pharmacy, I was finally going to get the help that I needed. I began to go to Alcoholics Anonymous because I was forced. Like we hear about all the time in AA, I was not interested in sobriety and all that stuff. I just wanted to stop being in pain and getting in trouble.

In AA, I got so much more than I bargained for. I got a sponsor because that's what I was told to do. I had no idea what I was getting into. I started working the steps. My first sponsor didn't have a car so I had to pick her up and take her to meetings everyday, which was awesome. It was exactly what I needed.

Even though I was going to AA, I was still drinking. I really felt because my drug of choice was hospital pharmaceuticals that I could still drink alcohol. So I actually drank the first three months I was in AA and then stopped. I do not beat myself up for that because that's what so many of us do.

When I was out of work as a nurse new to recovery, I worked in a deli and for UPS. I also worked helping a friend of mine clean swimming pools. In the beginning of my recovery, I was doing completely non-nursing jobs. I was being monitored and, eventually, got my nursing license back.

When I had about a year in sobriety, I went back to work in a hospital setting through an agency. This was perfect because, as an agency nurse, I was not allowed to hold the narcotic keys. I also got to set my own hours so that I never missed my home group, my other meetings or my Caduceus meeting.

I still remember the first time that I had a needle and syringe in my hands in sobriety to draw up Demerol, which was a drug I hadn't even liked. That was the first time I experienced what I now know as "conditioned withdrawal." I had a very profound physical reaction just by drawing up the Demerol and got physically sick. I wish somebody would have warned me about that beforehand.

I continued to work, being very careful giving medications to patients, when one day I was floated to the emergency room. I felt I was ready for this, even though I knew I might run into "C," a nurse manager in the ER who had been a party to that terrible intervention at my previous job when I was fired.

At this point, I was very involved in my recovery, working the steps and going to meetings all the time. I felt if my seeing "C" was meant to be, it was going to happen. Although I was not going to go out of my way to avoid her, I wasn't going to try to run into her either.

On this particular morning, the ER was very busy and when I turned the corner, I almost ran right into her. She was taller than me and when I looked up into her face, I saw she was not happy to see me. I looked her right in the eye and said, "You can ask me anything you want. A lot has changed in the past year." She said, "No. No, that's OK."

My agency called early the next morning to tell me that the ER didn't need me, which I knew wasn't true. I knew they needed extra nurses. Later on "A," my boss at the agency, called and asked me what happened at my last job, saying, "I want the truth." It was obvious that "C" had called and was causing trouble.

I had worked so hard to do everything to get back to work, so the truth just flew out of my mouth. "A's" response to what I said was "That b----." So "A" went to bat for me with the hospital and fought for me to work there. "A" revealed to me later on that she was in recovery, too.

In spite of that, I was still banned from working there, so all the discrimination we hear about nurses receiving in monitoring programs isn't always "newcomer paranoia." There is definitely discrimination out there. But the rejection made me stronger. The rejection was God's protection: I just wasn't meant to be at that particular hospital's ER.

In hindsight, I can now appreciate that perhaps "C" has only had negative experiences with addicts or alcoholics. At the time, I was devastated that someone would be so spiteful, but I have learned in my recovery that "hurt people, hurt people." She was obviously suffering from something and it did not pay to be angry at someone who was sick.

Back then I was told "Guard your anonymity with your life." I did what I was told to do, although a few key people knew my story. It was because of "A" advocating for me that I ended up working at another ER. This new ER was awesome. I loved it there so much that I ended up taking a position there. Since I was no longer working as an agency nurse, I kind of lost touch with "A" at that point.

Months later, my phone rang late at night with "A" sobbing that she had relapsed and did not know who else to call. This was my first real Twelfth Step call. Had I not been forced to divulge my history to "A" all those months ago, she would not have known who to call. It was amazing that she was initially the one advocating for me, and now the tables were turned.

Being a sober nurse working the night shift in that ER, I got to twelve step a lot of patients. I even ran into sober people who you can spot because they speak the lingo or wear something like a medallion.

I remember one patient in particular who was having an acute MI. When I pulled up his gown to put the EKG leads on, I saw the medallion with the circle and the triangle, which is the symbol for AA. I just whispered in his ear, "Are you a friend of Bill's?" When he said, "Yes," I just winked at him and said, "I take good care of his friends because I'm one, too." You could just see the relief on his face. There are so many little stories like that and it is always by the grace of God that I get to see these things because my eyes have really been opened.

Eventually, I got burned out in the ER and decided to go back to school. I started applying to anesthesia programs even though I knew nothing about the profession except what I saw in the ER. I knew that nurse anesthetists responded to our traumas and our codes. They also did our intubations and lumbar punctures when the ER physicians couldn't get them, but that's all I knew.

164

I moved to another part of the state to attend an anesthesia program. Until I was a senior anesthesia student, nobody had ever asked me on any applications for school or anywhere else about my history. That's when I was asked all those questions I didn't want to answer on an application to receive a stipend. Questions like, "Have there ever been restrictions on your nursing license?"

At this point, I had about six years sober and was still going to AA and doing everything I was supposed to do. I got really scared because I was a senior and well on my way to graduating. I was afraid to lie and afraid to tell the truth because I'd been screwed for doing both in the past.

As fate would have it, somebody was looking out for me because the physician who was to do my physical exam for my clinical rotation called in sick. This meant I got to take the application home and I called my sponsor. Then I called the American Association of Nurse Anesthetists' hotline and told the peer assistance representative everything. She was extremely helpful. She called my anesthesia program director and gave him a hypothetical situation, asking him how he would handle it if he had a student like this. Of course, he said he'd be very supportive and then she told him, "Well, this is one of your students."

I was instructed to call the director of the anesthesia program at home, which was something no student wants to do. As it turned out, he was out when I called, so I had to call back again at ten o'clock that night. Again, as fate would have it, my home group was that night. So I shared about all this at my home group, came home and called him. Here I was, just dreading making this phone call, not knowing how he was going to react.

Although he was unbelievably supportive, the director said, "Well, it looks like you are not going into clinical tomorrow because we need to talk about this." My stomach just dropped as all those old feelings came up, like "Oh God, I really blew it this time."

I had already established the reputation of being a good student, who was very reliable, dependable and prepared. I took the work very seriously, so the next day when I went into school he was really very kind. When the associate program director who was known for being a ball breaker joined us, she actually embraced me, saying, "I never would have thought it was you."

Really blown away by their support, I told them exactly why I was afraid to lie and why I was afraid to tell the truth. They both helped me fill out the application. They helped me come up with a statement that was categorized as "To Be Kept Confidential" where I explained all those "Yes" responses to questions I was afraid to answer.

Today, even though it's years later, I keep this statement updated and still use it. It describes everything I've done in the monitoring program, including the drug screens, monthly reports and everything I've done for my recovery, such as AA.

Back then, though, I handed the confidential statement in with my heart pounding because it was the first time I had done it. I told the person I handed it to that I would like the document kept confidential. I remember the woman glanced at it, said, "No problem," and threw the paper in a drawer without even reading it before locking that drawer. So, there it was. I was out of the closet and it was not a big deal.

Later on, I gave a peer assistance presentation which was the first time I broke my anonymity in front of non-recovering individuals at a podium. We had three classes of students in the room because the anesthesia program was two years, plus a semester. I just basically told my story at this "Brown Bag Seminar" after hanging up the Twelve Steps and Twelve Traditions posters I had borrowed from my home group. The presentation was very well-received and a couple of people even cried.

The experience I had in school really helped when I went looking for a job after graduation from the nurse anesthesia program. By then, I had seven or eight years of recovery and was able to hold my head up. I was no longer ashamed of who I was because I knew I never would have chosen to have this disease. It just happened.

I flew out west twice to interview for nurse anesthetist positions. On three out of four interviews, I was hired right on the spot, even after disclosing my entire history. I was very impressed with the support I received and was embraced for my honesty. The chief anesthetist who actually hired me couldn't stop crying. I later learned that one of her best friends was a CRNA who had just died of a drug overdose because she had been diverting.

Moving cross-country and working as a new CRNA took some major adjusting. Finding new meetings, a new sponsor and plugging into AA out here took an adjustment. As a student, I had gotten involved with AIR, Anesthetists In Recovery, an online group which is equivalent to a closed twelve step meeting for anesthetists. Through AIR, I was told who to get in touch with when moving so I was able to contact local peer assistance after I got settled.

Due to my involvement with AIR online, I was chosen to be a national advisor, which blew me away. It was like so many years ago when I asked somebody to be my sponsor and, later on, when I applied to the anesthesia program: I really didn't know what I was getting into. But I said "Yes," and just did it.

It has been absolutely incredible, getting hotline calls from all over the country and speaking nationally. It is a daily commitment which is exactly what I need. Every time I speak it is very liberating. It feels good letting people know that there is a solution because I still remember being in the pit of despair, thinking that there was nobody else out there like me and that I was the only one doing this. I felt so alone and so ashamed because I knew what I was doing was wrong, but I just could not stop. Later on, I found out it's a disease.

So, now when I get calls, I tell nurses, "You're not a bad person, but a sick person who needs help." I truly wish that there would have been someone like that there for me, although things worked out fine for me because I had the detective. Yet there was nobody in nursing who helped me and we can do better than that.

It is really important that we take care of each other and help one another instead of being content, saying, "Nurses eat their young." As the saying goes, we have to stop "circling the wagon and shooting inward."

In recovery over fourteen years now, I just went back to school for the second time in sobriety to pursue a PhD. My doctoral dissertation will most likely be on the phenomena of cue reactivity, which is what I experienced years ago when I drew up Demerol that first time in recovery. This has never been looked at in nurses or CRNAs who have taken drugs from the workplace and who must be able to deal with these cues after return to work on a daily basis.

Employers often don't want to hire nurses in recovery because they don't know how to do it. If they don't do re-entry safely and effectively and the person relapses, they say, "See. I told you I shouldn't hire this person."

Re-entry should only be done when each and every precaution is taken. People need to appreciate that even then, there are no guarantees. On the flip side, employers do have non-addicted nurses who might start diverting and are often among the least suspected individuals, so this black-and-white thinking about who has a problem has to go.

Having a solid foundation in recovery, going to Caduceus meetings and having full disclosure and support in your department is really important. The AANA also recommends random drug testing, a back to work contract, taking naltrexone and NO practice in anesthesia for a minimum of one year after re-entry.

In my opinion, it is also important for nurses to have gone through all twelve steps or, at minimum, the first five steps before re-entry into nursing. There is a head full of anger, self-pity, resentment and fear before the nurse in recovery completes the fourth and fifth steps. A head full of such negativity, when combined with a fistful of fentanyl, is a recipe for disaster.

While I believe we have made progress and come a long way, there is still a lot of work that we need to do. I hope in the future to help set gold standards for education, intervention and re-entry in nursing and feel very privileged to be a part of that work.

"Go Straight! Go Straight!"

While I was never given the playbook on life growing up, I never thought this would happen to me; never in a million years. I certainly didn't go into nursing to get drugs.

My parents drank alcoholically, although they never drank before five o'clock and always got up for work the next day. As a teenager, I couldn't have friends sleep over or anything like that because I never knew what it would be like at home.

Many times I would come home from being out with my friends to find my father passed out in the chair, or on the floor. Because I knew they were alcoholics from a very early age, I swore that would never be me.

As long as I lived in my parents' home, I never really drank. I was the designated driver because I didn't even like the taste of alcohol. My cousin struggled for many years with drugs, so I knew the dangers of that, too. I wasn't a stupid teenager. I knew it ran in families.

I graduated nursing school and immediately started working in pediatrics. I loved my job from the beginning, but it became my only identity. I worked nights, so all my friends worked while I slept, and I worked while they slept. I became very lonely and didn't have any other support system because of the way my parents were.

I started having pain. I can't say when it happened exactly. We used to go home with left over medications. You name it, we came home with it. We really didn't think twice about it. Wasting was such a lax thing on my unit because we trusted each other. Nobody ever thought that one of us would do something inappropriate.

When I was being trained on nights, and even on days, I was told since you are only giving a half a milligram of morphine and cannot take out less than two milligrams, you should hold onto the rest because if you have to give the patient more they won't be charged for another whole dose. So, I'd go home with morphine vials that would just sit on my desk and I'd never remember to bring them back and throw them out.

I don't know whether I took it for pain or sleep first. It was probably for both. For quite a few years, it was an every now and then sort of a thing; definitely not a habit from the get-go.

I worked on nights for six years, which was a very long time. I remember praying to God for this one patient like I had never prayed for any other child. I prayed that this one kid would get a break. And he did, or so it seemed. He had come in with stage four metastases. Even the oncologist, who never gave up on anybody, told us he didn't think we could save this one.

So I was shocked, yet delighted, that the chemotherapy shrunk the tumor immediately. They did surgery and he went home. This happened maybe a year or so after I'd become a nurse. Then, three years later as I hit my four year mark as a nurse, this child came back in with a brain tumor and passed away. I was so upset. I felt God totally betrayed me. By that point I was already burnt out.

At that time, I really did start using medication for emotional pain more than anything else. Things also got blurred with my drinking. When you work nights, it's not uncommon at the end of the shift to go to the diner as a group and get a screwdriver or whatever. After all, we'd worked a hard night, so in my head it was no different than anyone else who goes home after a hard day and has a couple of drinks.

In addition to that, though, I had friends calling me when they got out of work to meet them for Happy Hour at five in the afternoon, after I'd just woken up. I'd go to a bar and drink with them, because that's OK too.

Then there were times I was unable to sleep during the day, so I'd have a couple drinks. I think that's how it really became a problem with me. Getting blasted, just so I could get to sleep and forget. So it seemed like all of sudden it was OK to drink at night, it was OK to drink to forget and get some sleep, and it was OK to drink right after waking up.

There came a point where morphine wasn't cutting it for me anymore. I could take eight milligrams of morphine and it would do nothing. So, after this kid died and I'd lost any faith that I had, the pain was too much for me. The friends that I did have were never around because our schedules conflicted so much. My parents and my family did NOT want to hear about work anymore as that had become all I ever talked about. And there was nobody else to turn to for support.

So the only thing I had to kill the pain were the drugs I had sitting on my dresser. They didn't knock me out, but they eliminated the pain. They numbed me, and that's what I wanted. I did not want so much to be passed out. I just wanted not to hurt anymore.

I never denied my patients their pain medication – ever. They always got what they were supposed to have. But if they were getting one milligram, instead of taking out a two milligram vial, I'd take out the eight milligram vial. It got to the point that I was taking as much as I could get.

Eventually, I needed morphine every day. The times were getting closer and closer together and I just couldn't take out

172

as much as I needed because I didn't take it out unless a patient needed it. So I started drinking more and more. I told myself I wasn't a drug addict because I didn't do drugs every day and I told myself I wasn't an alcoholic because I didn't drink every day. Yet, there was never a sober day for me.

I justified myself because I was not the street drug addict; mine were the clean drugs, pharmaceuticals. And alcohol's not illegal. I remember buying two one-gallon bottles of vodka and then, a couple days later, going to a different liquor store because I didn't want them to think I was an alcoholic, which is pretty ridiculous when you think about it.

My use eventually caught up to me. I switched to Dilaudid because I couldn't get the effect I needed from the morphine anymore. It took a lot less Dilaudid for me to be able to achieve the same effect or feeling, which actually was a non-feeling state.

One day, one of the nurses questioned why I'd taken out the higher dose vial as opposed to the lower amount. I guess she really didn't buy my excuse. I found out later my colleagues spent that weekend watching me and noticed I never got rid of any of the vials I took out. They didn't say anything to me but told the assistant nurse manager, who reported this to my nurse manager.

It was a Wednesday I will never forget as long as I live. I was told it was necessary for me to come in on a "patient care matter." I knew right away there was a real problem because you never get called to come in on a day-off about anything like that. That just doesn't happen.

I remember standing at my bedroom closet thinking what does one wear to be fired, because I knew I was going to be fired. I decided it didn't matter and went in to the hospital in jeans and a tee shirt. I didn't need to get all dressed up to be fired.

As they grilled me, I denied what they were saying for about a half-hour. I just kept saying, "No, it wasn't me. That would mean I'd lose my license." I admitted being an alcoholic, but I did not want to admit being an addict. I mean, for God's sake, an addict? The stigma of admitting that was too great for me. An alcoholic's bad enough; but an addict?

As they were pushing me to admit I had a problem with drugs, I remember thinking to myself, "I didn't really do this. I did not REALLY do this." And I kept denying it, until my nurse manager finally said, "Well, if it wasn't you, then it must be this other nurse." I couldn't let that happen. I couldn't take another nurse down, so I confessed.

The supervisor for maternal child health, who'd known me for thirteen years, said, "Were you taking it for someone else? Maybe you were giving it to somebody else?" In her mind that would be far better than the fact that I myself was an addict. But I was taking it just for me because addicts don't share well.

Human resources told me a whole bunch of things I didn't comprehend at the time. They handed me a pamphlet, saying, "You should contact these people," which turned out to be the peer assistance program in my state.

I remember being asked if I needed anything from my locker upstairs, but, at that point, all I wanted to do was leave. My humiliation, devastation and shock took over. So I just took the pamphlet and left, truly devastated.

It was as if somebody had told me all of a sudden you're

174

homeless. Life as I knew it was gone. The only thing in my life in which I had any pride was my nursing. I had completely lost who I was. There was no "me" anymore. I was just "the nurse." In fact, when I'd meet people, though I'd say my name, it was automatically followed by, "I'm a Nurse." That was who I was; and being a nurse was, truly, all I was.

I remember coming home, looking in the mirror, and thinking to myself, "How did this happen?" Then I just crumbled, sobbing, because I had no idea what to do now. How was I going to tell my parents? How was I going to tell my friends? How was I going to support myself?

I figured I would sell my apartment, take all the money, do a whole bunch of drugs and kill myself off that way. That idea seemed far better than having to let anybody know what happened. I thought I would lose my license altogether and that would be it. I didn't know anything about peer assistance or monitoring programs at the time.

I called the number in the pamphlet that Wednesday and then I had to wait until Monday to meet the person I spoke to. I still remember that first interview, however, those were five very long days waiting for Monday.

For the first two days, I abstained from everything, all alcohol and drugs. My bones hurt so bad. My head was pounding and I was in so much pain. It was the first time I ever understood what people meant when they said that their hair hurt and their skin crawled. I ran a fever of 103. I was vomiting and having diarrhea and everything else under the sun.

At that time, my friend happened to call and asked what was wrong. I made the mistake of telling her what had actually happened. She lives over two hundred miles away in another

175

state and came up that day. She's a social worker and told me I had to tell my parents. She also told me I could not detox in my apartment because I might have a seizure. I said I was absolutely not leaving.

I am not at all a violent person by nature, but when she told me that, if I didn't go, she would call the cops, I threatened to throw her out my window. Of course, it is a first floor apartment, so I'd have ended up throwing her about two feet to the ground, but the threat was there. Now, years later, I am able to chuckle at all this, but what I said to her then was said with such venom.

She continued to insist that I needed to tell my parents. So, shaking up a storm and ready to have a heart attack, I called my parents. My mother said to come over, so we went. As soon as I told my parents, as soon as the words were out about what had happened, my friend the social worker left. After I told them everything, my mother suggested I sleep over there, and I agreed.

It was then that my parents made their usual martinis, and my mother said, "I don't think alcohol was ever your problem." I agreed that my problem was the drugs. So when she asked if I wanted a glass of wine, naturally, I took it.

From then on, I drank instead of using drugs. I didn't realize until much later that the brain will pick up alcohol in place of opiates. I didn't know that at the time, but I knew I wasn't shaking anymore. In fact, I was feeling really good. So I continued to drink. You would think losing my job, having to surrender my license to the state, and not working at all, which caused great fear and humiliation, would be enough to make me stop completely. But it was also because of those things that I continued to drink.

Here I was, with no identity and no respectable income. When I ran out of vacation time and the hospital stopped paying me, my parents gave me money to pay my bills. Instead, I was using the money to buy alcohol. I was being drug tested eight times a month in an outpatient drug treatment program which somewhere along the way had gotten the idea that opiates was my big problem, not alcohol. So while they tested me for recent alcohol use, they weren't doing the ethylgluconide testing which would have detected alcohol use during the past three to five days.

My disease is smart. It allowed me to tolerate not drinking for twelve hours because I knew I could drink after that. I was able to go the twelve hours because I knew if I got caught, I would not be able to drink at all. So I got very good at scheduling my drinking around the testing.

For the first four months, I went completely undetected and I continued to drink every day. At this point, I was drinking a little over a liter of vodka a day. I was able to complete the three-month treatment program and continued going to one group and individual therapy session a week.

I came up on the radar twice for alcohol, but convinced my therapist both times that I drank because I wasn't ready to go back to work yet. He asked why I didn't just tell him that I was not ready to return to work, rather than drink.

I drove out-of-state to visit my friend the social worker. As I was driving back, though, I had a minor fender bender. The teens in the other car wanted to call the police. I knew that was trouble because I'd been drinking. I'd never gotten arrested for a DWI before this. I'll never forget this because it was the night before my mother's birthday.

177

By the time the police processed me, it was about two o'clock in the morning. Like a good alcoholic, my license had been suspended because of an unpaid parking ticket. Of course, my car wasn't registered, there was no valid inspection sticker and I'd also forgotten to pay my insurance because I was using the money to drink.

Due to all those things, the police refused to release me on my own recognizance. They set bail at five hundred dollars, but I had no credit card or cash with me. So, I went off to the detention center for what would be the next twenty-four hours.

The morning of her birthday, I called my mother from the detention center. To my horror, when the officer asked if she would accept a collect call from an inmate in the county detention center, she hung up. They called her number again, and the phone rang a lot. My father finally answered and I told him I'd been arrested. He asked where I was and after I told him, he said they'd be right down, but they didn't come. Instead, they called an attorney in the state I was in.

I didn't get out of detention for another fourteen hours or so. All the other girls there were in for robbery or assault with a deadly weapon. They were all very nice, but every single one of them had been under the influence of alcohol or drugs when they committed those crimes. Every single one of them!

This was the first time in a long time I had gone twenty-four hours without a drink or a drug and I saw that I'm no different than any of these other women. There was no difference; and that shocked me.

My next thought was that I could've killed somebody in that car. I put in danger the very population that I swore never to harm; the same exact population that I cared for. I had be-

178

come the person that I most despised. Whenever kids came into peds after being injured by a drunk driver, I thought what a horrible human being that person was. And I was that person. So I swore to myself that I would never, ever, ever drink again. Never.

While in detention, my parents called my therapist and told him what had happened. I was so angry when I found out what they'd done. I thought, "How dare they call him!" because the whole time I had been thinking, "I just won't tell anybody what happened." But the jig was up now.

When I got back home I was informed I had to see my therapist the next morning. I hadn't gotten back until two in the morning, so I had to see him eight hours later. Needless to say, my therapist was not happy.

I think the realization in jail of exactly what I'd become had started to set in. So when he asked if I was OK, I said, "I'm done now. I think I'm done lying." He told me that was good to hear. When he asked what happened, I told him, "I drank. What do you think happened?" I was so angry with myself that everybody else within my range was going to get my anger, too. When my therapist asked why I drank this time, I told him, "I never stopped drinking." The shock on his face was overwhelming.

Leaving my therapist, I came home. With my favorite liquor store in walking distance, I bought a gallon of vodka. In less than fifteen hours from the time I had sworn I'd never, ever drink again, I was drunk. That's when I knew I could not do it on my own and that I needed something else.

During my session with my therapist, he had pushed very hard for me to go inpatient treatment. I was undecided. My mind

179

was still just whipping around corners because that had really been the first time I had been twenty-four hours without a drink. I really didn't want to go inpatient. I was convinced I would be able to do it on my own but I knew, at this point, that I couldn't. That was my real "Ah-Hah" moment.

So I called him up and told him I had to go inpatient. He asked me to promise him that I wouldn't take another drink before I went, and I told him I couldn't do that. It took two weeks for me to get into inpatient treatment and each day I drank like crazy.

Every day, my mom would ask if I drank because she didn't want to believe I couldn't stop. If she called me at ten in the morning, I'd already been drinking. The day before I went into rehab when I admitted I was still drinking, my mother finally said, "I guess you really do have to go to rehab." She, too, had much denial about my problem.

When I went inpatient, I learned a whole lot about the disease, which was great. Being a nurse you'd think that I would understand the whole disease concept, but you don't somehow. You just don't. Nursing schools don't cover the disease model of alcoholism and addiction. They don't explain how it's the mammalian part of the brain that everything goes through and short circuits. We do not learn that the alcohol shuts off any kind of cognitive thought process. It was the first time I realized, "Wow! It really wasn't my choice." Like they say in meetings, "It's your choice about the first drink, but after that you no longer have a choice."

It's not that I could let myself off the hook by the disease concept, but the disease concept made it possible for me to understand better that I had to do A, B, C and D. I had to do certain things to stay sober and that trying stay sober on my own wasn't ever going to work.

Years later, I found out that the inpatient treatment staff really didn't think I was going to make it when I left there. They knew that my parents were picking me up and they'd had conversations with my parents. I warned the staff not to call my parents after five in the afternoon because they are not coherent by that time of day. The staff had made the mistake of calling after five o'clock and didn't like what they heard.

This is why the treatment staff was very direct in telling me that Alcoholics Anonymous is the only thing that's going to save me; that if I didn't go, I was going to die because I'd never stay safe on my own without any support system out there. They told me I had to build that support system myself and that I can't rely on my family.

That is primarily why they didn't feel I was going to make it. They begged me to take a train home because they didn't want me going home with my parents. I remember, when my parents came to pick me up, before we even pulled out of the lot, my mother said, "You know, AA is a cult." I'd learned enough by then, though, to say, "Yeah, but it's a good cult."

So, I left inpatient and went to my first AA meeting outside of rehab that night. I did ninety meetings in ninety days, as suggested. I did what treatment had encouraged me to do, which was to let people in the AA meetings know when I shared that I lived by myself. I had to tell them that I did not have a support system, so they would know to call me and look for me at the meetings. I did all that and it was a huge help. I was able to build up a very strong support network.

I couldn't read in the beginning of my recovery because I had

181

the attention span of a gnat. I would read one sentence and that was about all I could handle. So, having a sponsor was very important. My first sponsor taught me the basics, like when you're having a bad day, take a shower and start your day over again. She'd tell me to lie down, take a nap for a half hour, get up, take a shower, eat something, and start the day over. She suggested I eat something sweet when I had a craving or call another alcoholic before picking up a drink.

I remember about a week after rehab, I was at the intersection in front of my apartment complex. My apartment was straight ahead and my favorite liquor store was to the left. I called my sponsor while at that red light and told her, "My liquor store is to the left and my apartment complex is in front of me. If I go to the left God wants me to drink and if I go straight God wants me to go home." My sponsor gave me very specific instructions over the phone, telling me, "Go straight! Go straight! God doesn't want you to drink."

It was that simple a thing, but I really needed that voice outside myself to say, "Go straight! Don't drink!" because I had that voice inside my head saying "Go left! Go left!"

So I went straight – in so many ways! I kept going to meetings, got involved in my home group, took the cookie commitment for my group, got a sponsor, did my ninety meetings in ninety days, got my ninety day coin and worked the steps. I kept going to meetings.

People in my life said my former employer was going to ask me to come back because I was a great nurse. The people I had worked with kept saying they thought it was the hospital's fault because I always got the half-dead patients and I did so well with them. No matter what difficult patient came in, they always gave them to me because they knew I'd take good care of the patient. One of the nurses I'd worked with even called me up and said, "You have to come back. They're giving me the patients they used to give you - and I can't handle it."

When my former employer called me one day and asked if I would come back to work, I was shocked. When I met the nurse recruiter, she said, "I am going to be straightforward with you about this: the fact of the matter is that you were a really good nurse and we need you back." To me, that was a testament to how much better I could be without alcohol and drugs than what I was like while drinking and using drugs.

I was just about six months sober when I returned to work and about one week shy of the day I had gotten fired a year earlier. I had to go back on the day shift, which was fine, but it was so odd going back. Up to that point, I had not even driven down the road that passes the hospital because of my humiliation about what had happened. So, when I walked in, I felt at any moment the police were going to arrest me for being there.

My first day went well. They had me follow another nurse who showed me the paperwork and things like that. Nobody really gave me a strange attitude. I cracked a couple of jokes about my situation because I wanted coworkers to feel comfortable talking about what happened with me.

The second day, my therapist from the drug treatment program came in for a "back to work" meeting with myself and the staff. He explained about addiction and alcoholism. I explained I'd cracked jokes even though I didn't find any of this funny because I wanted them to know I had spent nine months crying over this, and it's time to stop that. I told them I wanted them to feel comfortable coming to me directly and asking me questions, rather than talking to each other behind my back and deciding the answers for themselves. There were no limitations on what they could ask me; and if I didn't want to answer, I'd tell them that.

This opened the door for questions. For the first three months, there were lots of them. A few told me that people had said I had worn long sleeve shirts because I was trying to hide track marks. This cracked me up because I never had track marks on my arms.

While I was glad I went back to work and I loved it, I was being watched constantly, which was difficult. In the beginning, I couldn't simply have a "bad day." People kept asking, "Is everything alright? Is there something you want to talk about?" If I was tired or just having a bad day, people would tell me I seemed upset about something.

One day after I returned to work, my nurse manager called me at home and basically told me the same thing she'd said before when I was confronted. This time, though, I told her I'd be there in an hour. I wanted to prove to her I could be in there right away, that I wasn't doing anything wrong, and wasn't drunk.

When I walked in, she had this look on her face and, like the last time, said, "I think you know why you're here." I said, "Either I'm here because you're going to tell me I need to fix my documentation and you're firing me, or I'm here because you're going to fire me because of my documentation."

In my mind it couldn't be anything else. She could not be thinking I was doing drugs or drinking because, to me, it's so obvious I am not. I started to cry and she said, "My concern here is for you. Are you OK?" I explained to her how I really feel – that if I don't have my sobriety, I have nothing. That if she needed to fire me, I would keep my license and find another job; but if I ever lose my sobriety, I lose my license, and I probably won't get my license back or another job. But the worst part about losing my sobriety would be that I would lose me – again.

After I said all that, with tears pouring down my face, she asked, "Don't you feel better now?" I couldn't believe it! Do I feel better? I remember just thinking, "God, no, I don't feel better, but maybe you do!"

Soon back in the swing of things, I was back to getting those difficult patients like before but I had to be so much more careful this time. I couldn't risk losing myself again and there had to be that separation between me and my job. Because I knew that, I went directly to an AA meeting after my shift almost every day that I worked. Never on-time and always in my work clothes, but I was there at the meeting.

I was taught that anonymity is not towards each other in the rooms of AA. Anonymity is at the public level, but we should know each other in the meetings. The guy who taught me this said, "If I get sick and go into the hospital, how are you going to find me?" I realized that he was right, and, when I really thought about this, I realized that I knew almost everyone's last name and occupation in the meetings I attended regularly.

Other people thought I really shouldn't break my anonymity about being a nurse when I share, but when done in the room, it is not at the public level. I can't tell you how many times a nurse came up to me after I shared at a meeting and said, "Thank you. I really needed to hear what you said." We do need to know that we're not the only one; not the only nurse.

There was one guy I'd see in scrubs all the time, never knowing for sure exactly what he did. After I shared one night, he said, "Oh, I work in pediatrics too. I'm so glad you shared because I brought somebody here from work tonight for the first time." The other nurse was crying and thanked me so much for what I'd shared.

To be able to help somebody else is so important. That's one thing I got from going to the nurse peer support group meetings. It helped me see I wasn't the only one and that there was life after license surrender.

Some people at work are surprised I still go to AA meetings. I was back to work less than a year when my assistant nurse manager, of all people, said, "Aren't you done with that stuff? Didn't you do the twelve steps yet?" So I informed her that you kind of keep doing them and keep going to meetings.

The nurses at work who have become really friendly with me know that Wednesdays and Saturdays are my home group meetings and I make a concerted effort to get out of work on time those nights. They know I have to go and just say, "Go. Go on."

The people in AA have become my support system. The longer I'm sober, the more I realize that I can't rely on my family, because they don't get it either. My own brother who went to one of the family sessions when I was in treatment just asked me the other day, "Are you still doing AA?" And he's been educated about this disease!

Nurses sometimes ask me when I'll stop "going to that Alcoholics Anonymous thing." I just tell them the truth – I can stop going when I want to stop being sober. These are nurses, in the medical field, who are supposed to know about diseases. Yet they have no understanding that the only way

186

that this disease stays in remission is by taking our medication, which is our meetings.

At work once we were expecting an admission to come in, which was supposed to be my patient, but we found out that an oncology patient in sepsis was coming in all of a sudden. My nurse manager, the same one who had confronted me for drug-use, told me she wanted to give me the oncology admission instead of the other patient because the oncology admission was a lot sicker.

In my coworkers' minds, nothing had really changed. I was still competent, and, to a certain extent, they could still dump on me. So, I took the septic oncology patient. They continued to give me this patient for three weeks in a row. It got to the point after three weeks of caring for this patient that I knew I was going to be on for the next three days. Mid-shift, I realized, "I just cannot take this patient again tomorrow. I can't do this to myself again."

My grand-sponsor told me once, "When you have nothing left to give, you have no business giving what you have left." So I have to perform self-checks like this in sobriety. The excuse for always giving me the most heartbreaking, difficult patient, every single day I worked, was that I was so good with them. But because I take good care of patients does not mean it is therefore OK to suck me dry.

The reality is that my job is not going to protect me. I never thought of that before I got sucked dry, needed to go into rehab and went into AA. So I walked up to my nurse manager and just said, "I can't take care of her anymore. I'm really sorry, but I've had her straight for the past three weeks and I can't do it – she's sucking me dry." The nurse manager look-ed at me, and said, "OK."

For the next few months, I didn't get this heartbreaking case. Even knowing everything that happened to me and all I had been through, it seems that the solution for sick, difficult patients on my unit is to just suck me dry again. Though I don't think anyone saw it that way, it is my job to do self-checks in order to protect myself. They cannot do that for me.

Recently, I got certified in pediatrics, which was a big deal on my unit because I'm only the second nurse there to do so. They had a big sign up about this special distinction I'd received. Everyone asked how the test was and I told them it's basically what they already know. They asked if I studied and I told them I didn't. They then said, "Yeah, but you're smart."

All I could think of is what an incredible difference for me to go from being that alcoholic, that drug addict, that nurse everybody should watch, to the nurse that's smart and well-respected. Even the nurse practitioner who works with the oncology office told me, "I never worry when you take care of my patients because I know they're going to be OK. You'll think outside of the box in caring for them." I don't think anyone understands what compliments like that actually mean to me today.

My documentation isn't so hot. It may never be great, but I do keep trying to do better. I ask every now and then if my doc-umentation is OK. In my addiction, I wouldn't have cared about my documentation. I would've said, "Tough luck," be-cause I had too many other things to worry about.

I took care of a little boy whose father was a nurse. His son had been in the hospital about four or five days and I'd heard in report the father was really difficult and the kid was always uncomfortable. I wondered why we were only giving the patient Tylenol for pain.

188

Even though I have a very healthy fear of narcotics, I also have a very strong respect for what they can do when used appropriately. I understand parents are afraid of having their child become addicted and I work to educate them about appropriate use. So, I asked the father if he had any problem with us giving his son some Tylenol with codeine.

Since the father said it was alright with him, I medicated the child with it, as ordered. The kid perked up, and started eating and drinking. When the father said, "You are so what we needed right now," I almost cried. All I really did were simple little changes that, to me, were so obvious.

Even my nurse manager said the other day, "You know you're a real pediatric nurse." She wasn't talking about my recent certification. What she often tells me is, "Your patients are always very happy when I do rounds." And that is really what I am here for. That's the reason I became a nurse — to take exceptionally good care of my patients.

I Thought I Just Liked Drugs

I actually went into nursing school with the intention of going to anesthesia school. When I was fifty years-old, I entered anesthesia school, so my career in anesthesia nursing started fairly late in life.

Throughout college, I had a problem with alcohol but, for whatever reason, I recognized that was a problem. I have been abstinent from alcohol for forty years now and I think there are probably several factors associated with my ability to remain abstinent from alcohol all these years. The first was realizing that I had a problem and that I didn't drink like normal people. I would drink until all the liquor was gone and I had blackouts at times. For whatever reason, I recognized that was not normal.

The other thing that made it easy for me to stop drinking was that I married a woman who totally abstained from alcohol. We didn't associate with drinkers. Liquor was never a part of our life socially or in any other way, so it was just easy for me to stop drinking.

In retrospect, I've been an addict all my life or at least from the time I can remember. When I was in grade school, I had knee surgery. To this day, even though it's now many decades later, I can still remember how good it felt to have the intravenous narcotics for pain. At the time, I bragged to my friends what a wonderful feeling it was. Since that time, I have been trying to relive that feeling, or at least that's what I have been told.

I never thought of myself as an addict. I thought I just liked drugs because of the feeling they gave me. For some reason, I never made the connection with addiction. One of the biggest revelations for me in my recovery was that I am, in fact, an addict. That fact just changed everything for me. It told me that I was not just somebody who liked the feeling drugs gave me, but that I really did have an addiction disorder. This revelation allowed me to look at drugs in a totally different way.

I have never ever used a prescription for mind-altering drugs as directed. I have always taken them for the high. Even before I went to nursing school, I used to take my wife's medications for that purpose.

In nursing school, I continued my pattern and there were times late in my training when I would take patient medication for my own use. That pattern continued after I was licensed as a nurse and when I got into anesthesia school it continued. It wasn't an everyday thing, but there were a couple of incidents in school. One of the most memorable was when I overdosed. I had revived by the time the EMTs got there and remember congratulating myself because word did not get back to the school about it, so I wasn't dismissed. Imagine that! Congratulating myself, rather than recognizing that I had a problem!

Intermittently, the pattern went on after I graduated from anesthesia school. I would use occasionally and, of course, my use gradually escalated to the point where it was unavoidable that I was going to be discovered. I realized that and used to lie in bed at night, knowing that if I didn't stop I was going to get found out. I continued even though I knew what the consequences were going to be if I was found out.

At night while lying in bed, I would vow that I was going to stop using the next day. Of course, the first thing I did when I got into the hospital the next day was to get some drugs and abuse them.

It finally reached a point where it was impossible to deny the problem any longer. I'll always regret the trust that people put in me and that I betrayed. It is that trust which really allowed my pattern to go on for so long.

Once the problem was realized, I was terminated from where I worked. The hospital reported me to the nursing board but, out of desperation, I reported myself to the board before the hospital did.

I approached the peer assistance group with the American Association of Nurse Anesthetists and they directed me in what I needed to do and how I needed to do it. The nursing board in the state where I practice is what I would call an enlightened board with an alternative to discipline program. That program had the dual role of protecting the public safety while returning a trained provider into the workplace. They were kind, compassionate folks and I think they did a marvelous job with both tasks.

The first thing that was required of me was that I go away to a thirty-day inpatient treatment program. That was not an option. The board used the services of an addictionologist and I had to go for an evaluation because, initially, there was a thought that I would just do outpatient treatment. In hindsight, I think that would have been a mistake.

After I completed inpatient treatment for thirty days, I went through ninety hours of intensive outpatient treatment, followed by once a week follow-up for a year. The nursing board allowed me to return to nursing practice eight months after I entered the monitoring program. I had to put a practice plan together, which was really a recovery plan that had to be approved by the alternative to discipline program.

One of the items in the plan was that I had to be on naltrexone. Initially, I balked at that because I had now gone to the opposite end of the spectrum where I didn't want to take any drugs of any kind for any reason. But the board was insistent, so I went along with taking naltrexone.

I am very thankful that the board insisted on me taking naltrexone. Although I really believe naltrexone helped me, not everyone does well on it. There was some initial dysphoria when starting on it. Certainly there needs to be other things in place, too, but it allowed me to return to practice with a couple of advantages. First, the board felt comfortable with giving me narcotic privileges back right away as long as I was on naltrexone. This made it easier for me to find a job because I wasn't going to be restricted from giving narcotics.

The other advantage that naltrexone gave me I don't think I can ever describe adequately. Basically, what it did for me mentally was that I didn't have to worry about the temptation to use drugs. This was because I knew there was no upside to using. There was no high to be obtained by taking drugs while on naltrexone. This allowed me to get back into practice and to handle narcotics without a thought about diverting and getting high. I was able to get in the habit of safely handling the narcotics.

I initially worked in a hospital doing floor nursing for twelve months and was taking naltrexone during that time. Although I was allowed to return to anesthesia twelve months after I was discovered, it took me another ten months from that point to find an anesthesia job. So, basically, I was out of anesthesia for a total of twenty-two months. I continued on naltrexone for another six months after I returned to anesthesia practice and stayed on it for a total of eighteen months.

I have since stopped taking naltrexone and am comfortable without it. I think it is a tremendous tool in early return to work. If the board had insisted, I would have had no objections to taking it for the rest of my career. That would have been fine. In fact, there was a period when I had surgery and I spoke to the board about possibly going back on naltrexone. The board said it was my choice and, after talking with my surgeon, I decided not to go back on it. It turned out I did well after my surgery and needed nothing more than over-the-counter medications.

I have been clean and sober for four years now. I am back in practice for a little over two years and things are going well. I am happy and actually in a better place professionally than I probably was prior to my addiction. I'm chief of an anesthesia department which is growing and moving forward. I'm very glad to be a part of it.

I thank God for my recovery. I still go to 12 step meetings occasionally when I feel agitated, when things aren't smooth or if I feel I need to remind myself where I'm coming from. While I don't go to a physical 12 step program often, I am a participant multiple times a day on the online forum for anesthesia providers in recovery.

I am sure to go to a 12 step meeting anytime I read about the death of one of my colleagues. It's not so much because I'm afraid that I'm going to be the next one but to remind myself that this will always be an issue with me. I'll always have the potential, as does anybody. For me especially, the drugs will always, to some degree, be calling me, so I go to 12 step meetings occasionally.

Another huge factor in my life that has gotten me to where I am today in recovery is that I do believe strongly in a Higher

Power. I have always believed in one. I've always mentally known that there was a Higher Power out there and yet I never had that heart knowledge of the Higher Power.

During the early days of my recovery, that relationship was re-established with Somebody who's bigger than me and cares about me; who wants to direct my life and has my best interests at heart, regardless of what circumstances I may be put in. The circumstances may not be the ones that I want but I have to say that my Higher Power is looking out for me and directing me in a better way than I might be able to see right now.

That has turned out to be true a lot of times when I can't see what's going on in the midst of a crisis. Then I look back afterwards, and say, "Oh, yeah, I see." That's been another great big factor in this whole recovery process for me. I don't know that I've ever heard anyone say this but I really believe that the 12 steps are designed to put people back in touch with their Higher Power. I think that's the purpose of them – to get you not only sober, although obviously that's a part of it, but to essentially re-establish that relationship which will keep you in times of crisis. It guides my life, if I let it.

For me, it took thirty or forty years for prescription drug addiction to reach its full potential in my life. I believe with enough exposure it can really happen to anyone.

The Program That Saved My Life

I was the second child in a family of four children; or, as my mother put it, the oldest child in her second set of children since my brother was eight years older than me.

My mother was a nurse who graduated from a hospital nursing program and married my father right out of nursing school. At that time, married nurses were frowned upon so she was never able to practice as a registered nurse. Later on, she went back into nursing as a licensed practical nurse.

It was through my mother that I became aware of nursing. Often I went with her into the hospital where she worked with neurosurgeons in the operating room. Soon I became very interested in nursing as a career.

Upon graduation from high school in 1969, I was accepted into a university nursing program. It was in nursing school that I started learning to drink. I found out that if I went out to drink with my chemistry lab proctors, I could get a better grade in the lab.

My drinking increased throughout school to the point that when I took my state nursing boards, my room was the party room where all the beer was kept. I was able to pass my boards, but only with a very horrible hangover.

After I received my license, I started working as one of the youngest nursing supervisors in a local hospital. I was married to a man who was in the service, stationed in Korea. We tried to make our marriage work but ultimately could not.

During one of our attempts at reconciliation, I became pregnant with my first child. He was born with hypoplastic left heart and survived for twenty-nine hours. Upon being discharged from the hospital after his birth, I was sent home on meprobamate, or Miltown, as it was called. It was then that I discovered a way to cope with the stressors of life: by divorcing myself from reality with tranquilizers.

Soon I went back to work at the local hospital as a midnight supervisor. It was there on the night shift that I became aware that many of the other staff members were smoking pot. Occasionally I would show up after a four-day weekend very hung-over from partying on pot and beer.

Mainly to get away from the smoking and drinking routine, I decided to move to another state. Unfortunately, I continued to be immersed in the pot culture after I relocated. As an assistant head nurse on a very large floor, I tried to keep my partying contained to weekends but occasionally came to work hung-over. My staff would find a quiet place for me to lie down to help my "headaches." I worked there for two years before returning home because I missed my family.

Back home, I immediately went into the operating room to learn how to be a scrub assistant. It was there that I discovered Quaaludes, which helped me to sleep after long hours on-call. I also worked as an evening supervisor at the same hospital and often partied way into the night with my fellow co-workers after our work shift was over.

I moved to work at another local hospital where I started having headaches because I was constantly rotating from night shift to day shift, often in the same week. For headache relief, one of the neurosurgeons I worked with gave me a prescription for Valium, which worked even better with a couple of beers or some wine.

Next, I transferred to the OR in another hospital where, oddly enough, beer was kept in the refrigerator in the doctor's staff lounge. Sometimes we would drink a cold one after finishing up surgeries late at night.

My pot use increased when I married a coworker. His drug intake also increased and got to the point where I had to leave him when I discovered his IV drug-use. Taking my two children with me, I bought a house and tried to stay clean and sober.

It was at this point that I stopped smoking pot and only drank occasionally. I became pregnant and lost the baby at twelve weeks. Discharged from the hospital with a prescription for Xanax for my nerves and Halcion for sleep, I was soon using benzodiazepines to alleviate all stress in my life.

My drug-use increased with me spending longer hours at work. With sleep in short supply, I felt I needed to sleep whenever I wasn't working. Drinking now increased to include weekday drinking. I began going to the bars for Happy Hour with my coworkers and started having problems with the drinkers versus the nondrinkers at work.

As my drug-use escalated, I started having money problems as well. I couldn't remember what bills to pay and what bills not to pay. Eventually, I lost my house and moved into an apartment where my drinking continued to escalate.

Due to my increased drug-use, I became accident prone. At one point, I wrecked a bicycle that resulted in a broken leg. I drew quite a bit of criticism from my coworkers and family over that stunt.

Shortly after the disastrous bicycle wreck, there was a fire in my apartment. I was almost entrapped in the bedroom where I was asleep with the help of sleeping pills. I just barely woke up in time to get out of the house alive. I'm not quite sure what started that fire but I did lose all the possessions my children and I had. Two cats I loved dearly were lost in the fire, yet I managed to get out with my sleeping pills.

After that, I moved in with my Mom. Post-traumatic stress disorder set in at this point from being caught in the fire and with the help of concerned counselors, my medication use increased.

When my oldest daughter was turning thirteen a few years later, she experienced a suicide attempt. When she was discharged after a three month stay in a local psychiatric hospital, I asked her psychiatrist if he would detox me because I had become alarmed at the amount of drugs I was taking. I couldn't stop on my own.

He agreed, so I took a planned vacation from work and went in for detox and rehab under this doctor's care. Due to the large doses of benzodiazepines I was taking, I had seizure activity which required me to spend two weeks on the psychiatric intensive care unit hooked up to IVs. This meant that I was only able to spend two weeks on the rehab unit before my insurance coverage ran out.

Two weeks after I was discharged, I relapsed on even larger doses of medications. This time I was admitted only for detox since my insurance would not cover another rehab stay. A few short months after that, I was fired from my job of fifteen years at a hospital due to my poor work habits, which were a result of my drug-use and drinking.

I got another job working as a Director of Nursing at a nursing home and even though I vowed not to let drugs get me into trouble again, my drug-use escalated once more. My oldest daughter moved out the day she turned eighteen, saying she never wanted to see me again or even be associated with me. Meanwhile, my younger daughter was having legal issues due to smoking pot and running away from home. This caused her to be placed in state custody and she went to live in a group home for the next two years.

In 1997, I was accused of diverting medication at the nursing home, resigned from my position there and was reported to the nursing board. Two months later, I was arrested on charges from the nursing home and spent a week in jail where, oddly enough, I was allowed a prescription for Ativan to prevent me from having seizures. The charges were later dropped and, once again, I vowed to stop using drugs and alcohol.

With my nursing license suspended, I was given a chance to go before the nursing board for a hearing to tell my side of the story regarding the accusation of diversion. Since I was convinced at this point that I was never going to work as a nurse again, I did not even show up for that hearing. I just figured I might as well spend the rest of my life as a drug addict.

For the next six years, I continued to take my benzodiazepines and drink heavily. I even gave up driving due to seizure activity. It was during this time that my mother who had inspired me in my nursing career passed away.

One of my mother's dying wishes was that I return to nursing, so I stopped drinking and started concentrating on staying clean and sober. I did this by going to Alcoholics Anonymous and actively seeking out Caduceus meetings. The Caduceus meetings were hard for me to find but when I did find them I was welcomed. I found out that I was not alone. There were other nurses who had stories similar to mine and they were coping, working and living sober lives!

When I did reapply for my license, I was notified that it would be suspended for one year. Although my license was reinstated in 2007, I had trouble finding a job because of the length of time I had not worked as a nurse. But I had my license back! That in itself was a miracle.

Around this time, my youngest daughter was arrested on drug charges and her two young sons came to live with me. Having a three and a four year-old living with me didn't keep me from attending AA meetings, though. In fact, I found out that the children were welcome at most of the meetings I attended.

During 2007, I also started working with a certified addiction counselor. Clean and sober now, my oldest daughter who had said that she never wanted to be associated with me again, called and asked me to walk her down the aisle. Giving her away when she got married was one of the high points of staying clean and sober that year.

When I received my consent agreement from the Board of Nursing, I was very angry that the nursing board could tell me that I couldn't drink, had to go to meetings and had to provide urine specimens at their beck and call. I walked away thinking, "What gives them the right to impose all of these restrictions on me?"

It wasn't until I saw other nurses being monitored that I really understood that I had lost my right to do what I please when I descended into alcoholism and drug addiction. I had become a dangerous person. So, it was up to me to shoulder the burden of proof and show the board that I could once again be a responsible person.

To me, it's very much like when I was in nursing school because I had to show up for class. Now, I have to show up for meetings. In nursing school, I had to pass all my tests and now, I have to pass all my urine drug screens. In school, I had to complete all of my assignments and have them turned in before getting a passing grade. That's what I have to do now, once a month - complete my work, get my meeting attendance sheets signed and call my entire panel of counselors, physicians and supervisors to make sure their paperwork is submitted.

It is up to me to make sure that all of it is submitted on time. That equates to me completing my assignments so that I can be graded as a good nurse who has complied with the monitoring contract for that month. And, now, it's not such a chore. This is how I deal with those consequences: by proving to the nursing board that I am a responsible person and that I can be counted on again as a good nurse.

Currently I am working as a case manager for a monitoring organization that works with medical professionals who have drug or alcohol problems. This work reinforces my own efforts to stay clean and sober. It shows me what a struggle it is for everyone with an alcohol or drug problem. I am also studying for my certification as an addictions nurse.

As an advocate and active role model for nurses, my career objective is to promote reform in the areas of education and treatment. I see clearly that there needs to be a <u>big</u> change in the way that monies are earmarked for addiction and aloholism. This is an epidemic. It is a problem that is touching all our lives and we don't need to lose people the way I lost myself to alcoholism and drug addiction for so many years.

My last drug-use was in 2005 and I have not had a drink since February 22, 2006. While going to rehab taught me how to taper off medication without having seizures, my real rehabilitation started when I began going to AA and NA and working the program that saved my life. That's where my sobriety and rehabilitation took place – within the AA rooms. So, although I actually had the tools given to me in treatment, it took a long time for me to learn to use them effectively.

Sobriety didn't happen all at once. One or two days turned into one or two months; and the one or two months turned into one or two years; and now I am looking at four years clean and sober. Some of those days and months were very dark for me. Often, it was a minute at a time, but I held on. Now I honestly believe all of those old-timers who kept telling me, "Keep coming back," and "It works if you work it." They had the answer all along.

I have to work my program because my addiction works me. It wasn't getting me the places in life that I wanted and needed to be. It was only when I started working the program that it sunk in that this was the way I had to live. I had to change my life and use those 12 steps as a pattern for a brand new life. I honestly believe that is what saved my life and that is what has saved my nursing career as well. It has also made me a better nurse.

From Despair To Accomplishment

I grew up a very rigid Catholic in a small, rural town. My brother is eight years younger than I, so for a long time I was an only child. Both of my parents were alcoholics. My mother was a secret drinker while my father drank quite openly.

Though I didn't know or understand anything about the alcoholism I saw growing up, I was the typical child of alcoholic parents. I was very successful in school and didn't realize I was depressed.

My mother was a nurse who never worked because my father didn't want her to. She was basically a homebound person who seemed very unhappy to me. Looking back, I think she, too, was probably depressed.

At age seventeen, I was a nursing student. I finished one-and-a-half years of a two-year nursing program, obtaining all the clinical skills I needed. I went on to pass my LPN boards, but never worked as a nurse.

Instead, I married at age twenty and became a stay-at-home Mom. My husband and I drank socially and, over a period of several years, had four children. I was very successful, doing a lot of civic work in my community, although I wasn't ever able to practice my nursing.

During the fifteenth year of our marriage, my husband's alcohol use converted to daily drinking. It escalated and it got really out of control. This downward trend continued so, after twenty years of marriage, we divorced in 1980.

At that point, I started working full-time as an LPN. Going back to school for my RN, I did my college prep classes in the evening, worked during the day and raised my children. I did all the things I needed to do and graduated pretty much at the top of the class in 1986.

As soon as I passed my boards, I went to work in a long-term care facility for brain damaged infants where I had a wonderful opportunity to shine. As a charge nurse, I did a lot of education of the staff. I was also able to obtain a lot of technical skills, such as passing nasogastric tubes, inserting IVs and changing tracheostomies.

While working there for two years, my drinking began to escalate and I progressed to daily drinking. Without any consequences for my drinking, except that I was becoming really tired of getting up every morning and having to sober up to go to work, I tried my very best to stop drinking. I remember going to two AA meetings, but somehow I knew in my heart that it was not where I would be able to get sober.

At the time, I had also been using the diet pill phentermine, or Adipex. The combination of taking diet pills along with my drinking absolutely burned me out, both emotionally and physically.

Trying to be the perfect Mom, the perfect nurse and the perfect everything, I tried to break my drinking pattern by changing my routine. I transferred to the evening shift, which I thought would help me stop drinking, but it didn't. I continued drinking and using the diet pills, and I got very thin.

I became afraid to detox from alcohol on my own and felt that I needed to get away from my stash of alcohol and diet pills at home. Feeling I was spiraling out of control but still without any outside consequences whatsoever, I signed myself into a rehab in 1988.

Initially, to get the time off from work to go to rehab, I told my Director of Nursing that I was going on vacation. I explained that I wanted to visit my son in California for a month. As I was getting ready to leave on this "vacation," however, I told her the truth about signing myself into rehab. I asked her to seal my records so that no one would know where I was and she honored my request.

After completing rehab, I took a week off before returning to work. My second oldest child was getting her PhD in psychology at the time and she came back home to be supportive of me.

When I returned to work, I remember thinking I had planned everything to protect the story I had told my staff about going to visit my son in California. At the time, I had a loving staff who considered me a nurturing manager. When my staff repeatedly questioned why I hadn't come back from vacation with a tan, I had no reasonable explanation, so I finally told them where I had been.

My aftercare consisted of a twelve-week outpatient program. In addition, I was referred to a private therapist. She was a recovering ex-nun who opened a lot of doors for me. In particular, she gave me insights that allowed me to break through the denial I had - not about alcohol, but about life in general and the relationships I had with people.

A couple months after completing rehab, I was offered a supervisory position in a very large long-term care facility fairly close to where I lived. Before accepting the job, I told the Director of Nursing that I was in recovery. Even though drugs were not a part of my story, I chose to disclose my recovery status to her because I knew I would be in charge of the entire building, which included all of their controlled substances. The Director of Nursing was very understanding and hired me.

While my initial treatment saved what I call my "other life," the longer I remained sober, the more miserable I began to feel. I started to realize that something else was seriously broken in me that I didn't know how to fix. So, even more depressed in 1992 after being sober a few years, I received a diagnosis of dependent personality disorder and depression.

The combination of both diagnoses qualified me to receive full coverage through my health insurance for a twenty-eight day program for codependency treatment. While I had been going to AA, Adult Children of Alcoholic and Codependent Anonymous meetings prior to that time, I now shifted the focus of my recovery efforts into the CoDA and ACOA programs after my codependency inpatient treatment.

Although I'm a very spiritual person, I'm not necessarily religious in my behavior. Having steered away from the very strict Catholicism of my youth, my journey has been infused with miracles and people who have made marks upon my life. I do believe such things are God appointed marks on my life.

One such instance came along after I was working several years at the long-term care facility when I was given the opportunity to work per-diem at the rehab where I had gotten sober. Although I initially applied for an evening per-diem position, when I told the administrator that I was looking for full-time work in the field of addiction nursing, I realized that God was working a miracle for me, putting me in the right place at the right time.

I was unaware at the time that the interim Director of Nursing for the rehab actually hated addictions and the administrator had been praying for someone to turn that responsibility over to. After meeting with the administrator, I was hired on the spot to take over as Director of Nursing of the rehab.

The only drawback was the long commute of close to an hour. While going back to school for my BSN, the travel to the rehab facility became quite a strain physically, so I resigned after two years. I returned to work in long-term care facilities, completing my BSN and later went on to obtain my master's degree in addictions.

Over the years, I accepted several other employment opportunities in the fields of wellness and addiction, gaining much business as well as clinical expertise along the way. I went on to obtain advanced practice certification through the International Nurses Society on Addictions and other training, certifications and licensure as an addiction clinician in my state.

Several years ago, when my job as nurse manager of a detox facility was eliminated as part of a middle management cut that affected nearly two dozen other nurse managers, I came to the conclusion that I would never find another job working for someone else that would permit me to fully utilize all my skills in addiction nursing and counseling. Something kept telling me at the time to develop my own niche, which I did.

Receiving unemployment benefits, I decided to develop that niche into a business. So, about ten years ago, another nurse and I created a company which allows me to utilize all the skills I have developed over the years. The work we do keeps me in the trenches and I find it very fulfilling.

In addition, I began working in the area of nurse peer assistance in my state, performing evaluations and serving as a nurse peer support group facilitator.

I just completed all the requirements for my PsyD addictions. That was the only route I could take as there is no PhD specifically in addictions. My degree will allow me to integrate the medical aspects of addiction into my therapy practice.

When I needed to identify a clinical psychologist with a PhD to sign off on my doctoral studies, I asked the dean if my daughter, the psychologist, could be my mentor. The dean agreed to my proposal. So now, more than twenty years after my daughter took time from her own doctoral studies in psychology to come home and support me when I completed rehab, we are working together. Certainly working together, she as my mentor and I as her student, require good boundaries which we have been able to establish and maintain.

Looking back, my journey has been of one who has gone from despair to accomplishment. Now sober since 1988, I don't take my recovery for granted. While I do not go to as many meetings as I once did, the thrust of my recovery efforts is to continue recovering from codependency. That is what keeps me sober today.

Seemed Like A Good Idea At The Time

I think I have been an addict all my life. I can even say I was born an addict because, looking back now, I can see that the behavior was there. Of course, the drug-use wasn't there when I was a child, but the behavior was there, which I think was just a prelude to my drug addiction in future years.

I remember being the type of child who wanted the world to revolve around them. I was very egocentric, wanting my own way. That just plays into addiction because as addicts we are very self-centered. So I can see the behavior early-on, although it took some years for me to be able to look back and see it clearly.

I grew up in a household with an alcoholic. My father was a binge drinker and my mother was his greatest enabler. My father's side of the family had several alcoholics in it, so genetically I was fated for this disease.

My idea of what was OK was skewed from my early years. As a very young child, I remember seeing my father passed out on the floor, although I didn't know exactly what it was about at the time. I remember one incident in particular where he was passed out on the floor and I saw blood on the floor around his head. My mother just took me by the hand and led me around him, saying all the while, "Everything's OK. Everything's just fine." So my idea of what "just fine" meant and what "OK" meant was distorted from the beginning.

Growing up in an alcoholic home, especially with a binge drinker, was like growing up waiting for the shoe to drop every day. I never knew which would be the day my father would start drinking. Therefore, every day when I'd come home from school and open the door, I'd wonder if that would be the day he was home drinking.

Those days he was drinking would become several days of pure agony for my mother and I. Then he would stop, go back to work, and everything would be "normal" again. This went on for my entire childhood. Later, I found out that this went on during my sister's entire childhood as well, although she was many years older than I was. So she and I had the same childhood, but just at different times.

As a child going to elementary school, I always felt like I was on the outside looking in. I felt that I didn't belong, that I was different. I think this is very typical for people with addiction. It wasn't until later, when I actually got into recovery that I realized that this is how I felt as a child. It was only after I got into 12 step recovery that I felt a sense of belonging. That was the first time in my life I felt secure and safe with other people.

In high school, I experimented with alcohol a little bit, but was determined I'd never abuse alcohol because of my father's alcoholism. I also really didn't like it much, but it was something other kids were doing. So, I tried to be like them and experimented, too, but never really liked or abused it.

It was in my senior year of high school that I became engaged to the boy who lived across the street from me. Several years older than I, he had just finished college. Looking back on it now, I see that a lot of the decisions I made in my life fit into the category "seemed like a good idea at the time." I can see now that maybe some of these decisions weren't really that good. Many of my friends and my husband-to-be's friends at the time were getting married and engaged, although they were much older. So it was just one of those "seemed like a good idea at the time" moments for us to get engaged and we got married after dating a couple years.

At eighteen, I went into nursing school and remember once as a freshman having some kind of pain. The school nurse gave me a tablet. I have no idea what it was, but it was obviously mood-altering, because within twenty minutes I felt like I was on top of the world. I had never felt that way before. And I remembered that. Only an addict remembers their first high, although my addiction did not actually become active until years later.

My father had also passed away when I was eighteen. He passed away on Christmas Day and for several years after that, even though he had made my life and my mother's life miserable, the holidays were a very tough time for me.

About four years after he died and I had gotten married, my first son was born on December 25th. It wasn't purposeful; it just happened that way and that made Christmas OK after that. Shortly thereafter, our second son was born.

After I graduated from nursing school, I started working as an RN and had another one of those "seemed like a good idea at the time," which was to go to nurse anesthesia school. I had never abused any substances or diverted anything at this point and had never even thought about doing something like that.

When I went into anesthesia school, my husband essentially became mother and father to our sons because I had to spend so many hours studying, taking call, and doing all those things you have to do in anesthesia.

My reason for going into anesthesia was certainly not the best. I went into it because I wanted to make more money than a nurse could in those days. That was purely the reason I chose anesthesia as a career. It wasn't particularly for love of that type of work, because I never really did like it. It was a means to an end in terms of financial security and that was my reasoning for going into it.

After I graduated from anesthesia school, I started working as a nurse anesthetist. It wasn't long before I became really dissatisfied working as an anesthetist, but I'd gotten myself into this situation and didn't feel like I wanted to give it up. I didn't want to give up that financial security, so I stayed in anesthesia.

My husband got a job opportunity in the middle of the country, so we moved from the east coast. I got a job in our new location as a CRNA, where we lived for the next six years. A couple years after moving there, though, my husband and I had become distant. So while we were married for a total of ten years, we lived our lives as roommates for the last five of those years. We stayed together because of the children, but we finally decided that neither one of us were happy and separated.

It was an amicable divorce. Fortunately, we put the children first in terms of making sure that they were traumatized as little as possible. I stayed where we were living and my husband moved about three hours away. We made it a point that the children have as much time with their father as they could, spending many weekends and summer vacations with him.

Being a single Mom was probably one of the hardest times in my life. I was trying to be the single Mom, managing a household, trying to raise the children, and also working. So, after four years, I was pretty worn out and decided to move back to where I had grown up, to be close to my mother and sister.

213

Returning to my home state, I got a job in anesthesia. I still wasn't abusing substances, or even thinking about diverting anything, or drinking alcohol abusively.

Eventually, I started dating a man who was in training for a job with the government. After dating a couple years, my boys were becoming pre-adolescent and my oldest started having some major problems in terms of discipline. I'm not the best disciplinarian and wasn't good at controlling his behavior. As a result of our interactions, my younger son wanted to leave the house because he didn't want to be around us. This became a horrible situation that I just didn't know how to handle, so I tried counseling. Looking back now, I do not think that I gave it a good shot because my addict brain thought if counseling wasn't working right away, it wasn't going to work. So, I didn't continue counseling.

The situation with my son became so desperate that I finally called his father who by this point had remarried and moved further away from us geographically. He suggested I let my sons live with him and his wife. I really had to think about that. It was probably the hardest decision I have ever had to make in my entire life. I could see things were progressing very rapidly as far as disciplinary problems and that with two teenage boys it was not going to get any easier to deal with.

So, I made the decision to let them move to their Dad's. I have spent a lot of years feeling guilty and shameful about this decision and, still to this day, haven't gotten over it. Some members of my family pretty much shunned me during this time because they thought I was abandoning my kids. This got to me, too. Now that my sons are adults I know it was a good decision to have them move to their father's. As hard as it was to be separated from them, it was the best thing I could have done and was probably one of the better decisions that I made, though I really didn't feel that way at the time.

I continued to date this man and when his job training came to an end, he had to be transferred to a base in the U.S. I made a decision that since my boys were living with their Dad, that I would move in with my boyfriend to see how things went, knowing that eventually he would be transferred overseas.

So, after we moved, my boyfriend had a desk job for a year and I got a job as an anesthetist. I was still not abusing drugs. Eventually, he got an assignment overseas and we had to make a decision because I could not go with him unless we got married. So, another of those "seemed like a good idea at the time" decisions was made and we married.

The first few years were really wonderful. We had a great time and it was adventurous. It was different from anything I'd ever done. I didn't work overseas because it was expected that the wives would stay home and entertain to help their husband's career. So I did not work for a time as a nurse anesthetist.

The first place we were assigned was very cosmopolitan and wonderful, but the next assignment was the exact opposite. It was very impoverished. We had to take two years worth of food with us and had four hours of electricity a day. It was a tough, very difficult environment that we lived in for those two years. Everybody was sick from various parasitic diseases. There was also a coup while we were there, so we had to hide in our home for three or four days until that was over.

During the latter part of these two years, my husband's behavior started to change. He became somewhat paranoid, which is not too unusual for someone in his type of work but towards the end of the two years, he was getting worse. When we were offered a wonderful assignment in another foreign city, however, we said we'd go.

After we were transferred, my husband's paranoia escalated. It became all encompassing, to the point where he was not sleeping or eating. He felt everyone was following him and I did not know what to do. I felt that if I went to his boss, my husband would be fired, so I tried to manage as best I could. I was his only reality check, which was an incredible burden. Then, when he became more dysfunctional, I finally convinced him we had to talk to his boss. At that time, we were transferred to another country where he could undergo testing and then we were sent back to the U.S. for further treatment.

Back in the states, I went back to work in anesthesia with my former employer. My husband got much better on medication, but living with someone with this particular mental health problem was very difficult.

At this time my oldest son, who had turned eighteen, was becoming very difficult behaviorally. His Dad couldn't handle him anymore and asked if it was possible for him to come back and live with me. Of course, after all those years of guilt and shame, I said, "Absolutely he can come here to live." I was thinking I could make up for all the lost time.

Even though my husband was better when my son moved in with us, they didn't get along. It got to the point that each would come to me, complaining about what the other had done wrong. Of course, I allowed myself to be put right in the middle of that triangle and I tried to make everything OK. Growing up in an alcoholic home, I had to become the caretaker at certain points, so this fed into that piece of my personality. But no matter what I did, I couldn't make things

216

OK and I started having headaches. Every time I knew that my husband and son were both in the house at the same time, I would get headaches, which got progressively worse.

I continued working as a nurse anesthetist, primarily on an outpatient basis. The anesthesia group I worked in covered a lot of outpatient offices, so each of us were pretty much on our own. We would do the cases assigned in an outpatient office for a particular day and when we were finished, we'd go home. There was nobody around to cover for breaks or provide relief for lunch, so you just did your cases and then you were done for the day.

One day, I remember working in an ophthalmology office where cataract surgery was performed under sedation. There were nine cases that particular day, which was an incredibly long day. I had the worst headache I can ever remember having to this day. I made the decision that I was going to use something that I had at hand in my anesthesia repertoire to alleviate this headache because my head hurt so much. That was just my distorted thinking.

So, after the cases were done, I went into the bathroom and I used one of the medications that I had on hand. Within twenty minutes, my headache went away and my family problems went away. I was transported back to that first high I'd experienced as a freshman in nursing school. I knew I had found the answer and it was going to be OK.

That first time, I had used Demerol intramuscularly. It wasn't more than a couple of days later before I decided to use it again. I don't remember if I had a headache the next time I used it, but it didn't matter. Within a very short period of time, I went from using intramuscularly to intravenous use.

217

At this point, I was in my thirties. While I might have started using addictively later than most do, I hit the ground running once I did start. The only positive note about my use is that I never deprived my patients of their meds. I ensured that they were appropriately medicated and there was never any patient harm, though the potential was there.

My addiction went pretty fast after that and it wasn't long before I realized that I was getting into trouble. So, I went to my husband and said, "This is what you and my son are making me do. If you'd change your behavior, I wouldn't have to do this." That's how distorted my thinking was. Of course, this scared him to death and he went to my employer. Together, they both decided I needed to go into treatment.

Well, my mindset was that I didn't need to go to treatment. I just needed everybody else to change so I didn't have to do this. But they insisted on inpatient treatment and my boss finally said that if I did not go, I wouldn't have a job. So, I was forced to go.

The whole time I was in the treatment center, I was ticked off. I felt that I didn't belong there because I wasn't like "those people." But I did all my little assignments and all the things I was expected to do so I could get back to my job and get on with my life.

During that twenty-eight day treatment program, I was told by the staff that they had concerns about my going back to work in anesthesia, but I told them I'd be fine. My boss had said if I completed this twenty-eight day program, I could come back to work with no problem. Of course, my employer had no better understanding of addiction than I did.

So, I went back to work the same week I got out of treatment and, within just a day or so, I was using again. I was found out very quickly and fired from my job. Never having been fired before in my life, I was just devastated. I just didn't understand how this could have happened to me.

At this point, my husband's condition was under control with the mood stabilizers prescribed for him. My son decided to go into the military and my husband was offered an opportunity to go overseas again. Since I wasn't working because I'd been fired, this was another one of those "seemed like a good idea at the time" decisions. So, we went back overseas, where I was essentially a "dry drunk" because while I was not using, I was also not in recovery.

After leaving the U.S., my husband decided to stop taking his mood stabilizer medications. He became very sick again and I was sick in my own right, not being in recovery and just being miserable.

Quite frankly, I don't know how we got through those two years overseas. My husband became so paranoid he wouldn't talk to me in the house. We had to go outside because he thought the house was bugged. He felt everyone he worked with was working against him and when we got in the car he thought everybody was following him. He made all these paper lists, just like in the movie "A Beautiful Mind." It was just like that movie and it was just awful.

My husband decided during that tour that he was going to leave that job and ask for a stateside assignment, back to where we had been living in the U.S. He requested an assignment teaching at the training base and, when that was granted, we moved back to the states where I then got a job in a local hospital.

After my husband started teaching, he did well although he was still quite paranoid. For awhile I didn't use drugs, but after I was working about six months, I picked up again for no particular reason. Of course, I hadn't been doing anything to prevent picking up, so it really was just a matter of time.

I started using right at the same level where I had stopped before, which is what addicts do. Considering the medications I was using, it is just incredible that I used for a year-and-a-half at that particular job and didn't die. Occasionally, someone would ask me if I was OK, but I would just say I was tired or whatever, and blow it off.

During this time, my husband decided to leave his government job and go to school for architecture. I was going to support us at the time. So, he quit his job, applied to grad school and we moved to an area near the school.

I had interviewed at a local hospital where we moved to, which was a level one trauma center. I had never worked in a level one trauma center before and within just a few days of starting that job, I began using. Within four to six weeks, I got found out and was intervened on. Essentially, it was my CRNA supervisor and the anesthesiologist in-charge who asked me, "Do you have a drug problem?" Of course, I said, "No." They told me I had to give a urine drug screen, which came back positive, and not just for opiates because I was using anything I could get my hands on by that point.

Escorted out of the hospital, they reported me to the nursing board and the legal authorities. I went home and sat in my bedroom, with no idea what I was going to do. I was absolutely devastated. Even the term "devastated" does not describe what I felt. That was the one and only time in my life that I felt suicide might be a possibility because I didn't know how to stop using and I didn't know how to get help.

But I also remember sitting on the edge of my bed that night, looking up at the ceiling, thinking there has got to be some help out there for somebody like me. There has just got to be! And I really believe that was the beginning of my recovery because it's the first time I'd ever looked outside of myself to try to figure out what to do. It was the very first time I stopped trying to figure things out on my own.

Human resources and the Employee Assistance Program at work had directed me to go to a group called Caduceus. I had no idea what that was about, but it was a support group for healthcare professionals with substance abuse problems. The EAP also told me that I needed to go to treatment and told me exactly where I should go. When I went to Caduceus, they mentioned the same treatment place. Since I had been reported to the legal authorities, I also had a lawyer who just happened to mention the very same treatment place that my EAP and Caduceus had recommended.

All the signs were there and I was so beat down that I knew I couldn't do this anymore. I had finally become willing to listen to what somebody else had to say about what I should do. So, off I went to treatment.

When I got to the treatment center, there were about thirty people in the meeting room. I somehow knew instinctively that this was where I belonged. That's the first time I'd ever felt like I truly belonged somewhere. Here was a group of other people who were in the same place I was in and trying to do the same thing I was. We were all trying to figure out what to do with our lives and somehow I felt on some level, even as scary as it all was, that everything was going to be OK.

It was at this treatment center that I got it. I finally got an understanding of what was wrong with me. I'd felt for a very long time that because of the decisions that I'd made in my life that I was some sort of sociopathic reject or something. All I knew was that there was something wrong with me but I had no idea what it was.

While in this treatment center, I learned there was something I could do about my addiction. If I did the things these people told me to do, I could get better. Essentially, they were saying the same things that those people at the first treatment center said, but this time it made sense because I was open and willing to listen. I had become teachable at this point.

No matter what else happened, I knew when I left there after ninety days that I was going to be OK. I didn't make the decision right then, but shortly thereafter, that I would never practice anesthesia again. That was a hard decision to make but I just didn't want to have that struggle of walking into an operating room every day and being tested. I just didn't want to do that and gave up my CRNA certification. Of course, I had lost my license to practice nursing in the interim and had legal charges pending, but I wasn't fully aware of the criminal charges yet.

Since I couldn't work as a nurse after I came home from treatment, I had the time to really establish an incredible recovery program. I was able to develop a great network of people in Caduceus and in the 12 step rooms who essentially became my family. They got me through all those horrendous things like my matters before the nursing board and my relationship issues. I don't think I would've made it without that support.

I went to work in a little gourmet store for seven dollars an hour for the next two years. Those were probably two of the happiest years I can remember because I was doing something that I loved.

My husband was still very ill and we had no income, so he had to quit school. He had sold insurance in a previous life, so he got a job selling insurance. He had come to the family program when I was in treatment and one of the things that I had told him was that if he didn't take his mood stabilizer medication to stay healthy, I couldn't stay with him. He agreed to do that, but at a certain point I realized he had stopped his medication and he had started to slip back into paranoia again.

Although my addiction is not about him, I also knew I could not stay clean if I stayed in that environment. He became very resentful of what I had to do for my recovery and the network of people I'd established. He and I had become very enmeshed and codependent when overseas because we were pretty much all each other had. It was very hard for him to accept that I had to do things differently now to stay in recovery, so I eventually made the decision to separate from him.

Nine months after treatment, I was indicted on one felony charge for stealing drugs from the hospital. I was absolutely devastated. I thought that the criminal justice system had forgotten about me, but of course they hadn't. When I went to criminal court, the prosecutor recommended a sentence of three years in prison. I remember that the judge started to talk about her decision, but she stopped in the middle of what she was saying. My lawyer and I were trying to figure out what she was thinking as she looked down at her desk.

Then she just looked up at us and said, "No, I'm not going to do this. I'm going to take this under advisement for a period of three years. If you come back here in three years and have done everything you're supposed to do, I'm going to make

223

these charges go away eventually." I truly believe that her de-cision was Divine Intervention; that there was a Divine Hand in that decision. I was given a second chance.

That same week, I also had a hearing with the nursing board because I had reapplied for my nursing license. That was a tough week, meeting with the board and going to court. I took my sponsor and a couple of other people from my Caduceus group with me when I went to meet the nursing board. I was granted my license back but this was before the days of the state monitoring system that's in place now. At the time, you were pretty much responsible for setting up your own mon-itoring. I needed a nurse to volunteer to be my monitor and had to find a place to get my urine screens done. I also had to get documentation of the meetings I attended.

After I got my license back, I was offered a job at an addiction treatment center where a friend of mine worked. She offered to be my worksite monitor. Initially, I had restrictions on my practice, but these were all eventually lifted and my license was reinstated. This meant I was no longer required to be monitored, but I continued to go to meetings and do all the things that were suggested.

Two years after working in the treatment center, I was offered a job with an intervention program that was being established in my state to monitor impaired healthcare practitioners. I had heard rumors for years that this program was starting and was very excited about it. So, when I had the opportunity to work for that program, I jumped at the chance.

The contract to run this program started January 1st, and was for a five year period. Without question, this was the single most wonderful, rewarding job that I've ever had. I did a lot of education on impaired healthcare professionals and traveled throughout the state to speak to nursing, dental and pharmacy schools. I was finding out very quickly that there wasn't any education for medical professionals in the school curriculums on the disease of addiction.

We were able to assist a lot of people in my state to get the help they needed, monitor them to ensure they were safe to practice, and get them back to work. At the end of the five years, however, when the contract for this particular program went up for bid, we lost the contract to another entity. We were forced to close down, which was devastating because this was a team of wonderful people who I became very close to. It was a really tough time.

While this was happening, I had begun dating a man. After three years, we decided to get married, another one of those decisions that "seemed like a good idea at the time." I moved from where I had been working in the state monitoring program to a near-by state where he lived and practiced his profession.

I had become so caught up in my job with the monitoring program that I had slowed down on my meeting attendance. I also hadn't bothered to get a sponsor when I moved a distance away from where I had first gotten clean to take the position with the monitoring program. I had neglected everything that supported my recovery.

So, when I moved out-of-state and eventually married this man, it was just easier not to do anything. We lived in a very small rural area, where there were no meetings closer than a forty-five minute drive away. I had really convinced myself at that point in time that I was OK; that I really didn't need the meetings anymore; that I was doing fine and had no problem.

We went to Australia for a month-long honeymoon. It was here that I decided I wanted to have the experience of drinking an Australian beer while I was actually in Australia. I won't even try to justify this thinking or action. Looking back, it was inevitable. It was time for me to pick up again because I wasn't doing anything to prevent it. And so I had the Australian beer in Australia and over the next two years had an occasional cocktail or beer or glass of wine. I didn't really abuse alcohol, but I used it.

Still not going to meetings or doing anything recovery-related, I started looking for a job. I found a job at a local home health agency which was really the only job available in the vicinity. I started working and, almost immediately, when exposed to my drugs of choice, I picked up. I was off and running. The switch had been turned from "off" to "on" by the alcohol, but I hadn't had access to drugs until I got into home health. So, I hit the ground running again and began using non-stop.

This went on for a little over a year. I don't think my husband suspected until towards the very end. He later told me that he didn't know what to say or do, or how to help me when he did realize I had a problem. Eventually, I was intervened upon by my supervisor for diverting drugs and was reported to the nursing board.

The day after I was fired, I was in a treatment place outside of the state I lived in, once again feeling very ashamed, and humiliated. I can still remember that first day back in a 12 step meeting because I felt this tremendous sigh of relief when I walked in the door. I felt like I was home again. I was back where I belonged. It is a terrible place to be in when you are back out there using, knowing what recovery is because you know how good recovery can be; yet you just don't know how to get back there.

When I went to that first meeting, I knew I was back where I belonged. It was like getting back up on the horse again. I hit the ground running with recovery and just started absorbing all that I had been missing for so long. I successfully completed the treatment program and came home.

My husband drank and within the last two years of our marriage, he had started drinking excessively. I had talked to him about it while in treatment and asked him not to drink around me and not to keep alcohol in the house. Though he did not drink in front of me, he continued to keep alcohol around our house.

As my husband started exhibiting more alcoholic behavior, things became very difficult. He decided to run for an elected office, which added greatly to the stress. While I was trying to go to meetings and work on my recovery, he was drinking alcoholically, so it was a very stressful, difficult time.

Ultimately, my husband lost the election and I knew in my heart we could not stay together because of his alcoholic behavior. I hung on by my fingernails as long as I could because my ego didn't want to admit that I had "failed" again in a relationship. I knew he could no more give up drinking than I could stop myself when I was using. I understood that part, but also knew what I had to do for my own recovery. So, I moved back to my original home state.

Back home, I was presented with an opportunity to work at the same treatment center I had worked at years earlier. Because I had been reported to the nursing board, I had joined the monitoring program in the other state I had lived in with my husband and remained compliant with all they asked of me.

While with my husband, I had not been trying to find a job as a nurse because none was available in that rural area. Now that I moved back to my home state, though, I had to switch to the monitoring program in that state. This required me to become extremely humble because it meant I had to ask to be monitored by the very program I had helped to form years before. While this was a very humbling experience, by the same token, this was something that I knew I had to do to maintain my sobriety.

To this day, I continue to be monitored by this program and am very grateful for that opportunity. The way I feel now is that if I have to be monitored for the rest of my career, so be it. If monitoring is something that stays between me and picking up again, or helps prevent a relapse, then I'll just continue to be monitored. I feel that the more things I can put between me and a drug or a drink, the better. So, whatever I need to do to support my recovery, I'll continue to do.

I'm in recovery now for two-and-a-half years after previously being in recovery for nine years. I don't consider that time I was originally in recovery as wasted time, by any means. I feel like it was a foundation on which to build the recovery I have today. I am very grateful for every day that I am clean and sober.

I am also extremely grateful that I have been given another chance and I am trying to do it right, one day at a time. I am grateful for the program I am in. I have a job I really love today in a treatment center, working with people who are truly friends. I have a sponsor who I call every day and I'm doing step work. I will continue to do that work for the rest of my life, but only one day at a time.

Once Hopeless, Now I Am Full Of Hope

From my earliest memory, all I ever wanted to be was a nurse. I grew up in what I considered a pretty normal, kind and loving family. Very shy in high school, the very first time I was away from my parents was when I left home at eighteen to start college.

My first drink of alcohol was at a college party. I remember feeling very nervous, anxious and ugly at the time, but after my first beer or two, I immediately felt I had arrived. I had found the answer and began to develop a fast friendship with alcohol that initially was good, but then became my path to self-destruction as "our relationship" continued.

The nursing program at the college I attended was set up so that the first two years you took all your general classes and then you applied to be accepted into the nursing program. The first time I applied, I did not get in. My life-long dream came to a screeching halt at that point. I felt like the bottom of my life had fallen out, not because my family wasn't supportive because they were and then some, but because I did not know how to change to plan B. Although I was taking the steps to do that on the outside, my insides were crushed and broken. Watching my friends continue along "my path," without me, was difficult.

During the following year, my drinking escalated, yet, somehow, I was able to do well in class, raising my GPA and getting accepted into the nursing program. I was happy and my life was back on track.

The summer after my first year in the nursing program, I worked as a nurse's aide and fell, injuring my back. My family doctor started me on muscle relaxers and a pain med called

Darvocet. It was a magic combination, as it gave me the same kind of warm, floating feeling that alcohol did. I did not know it at the time, but a seed was planted. It was another fix for all the stuff inside of me that was hurting as much or more than the back pain.

As my back pain worsened during my last year of school, my family physician prescribed a stronger medication for me: Vicodin. I still remember the first day I took it because I had an out-of-body experience. Not only was there no physical pain, but all the pain inside me vanished as well, just like it did with drinking alcohol. That was the day I crossed the invisible line and I became an alcoholic/addict. Although I can see in retrospect that mood-altering substances became the center of my life, I did not realize this at the time.

By the time I graduated nursing school, it had taken me five-and-a-half years to complete the program. While I was elated to graduate, there was still a part of me that felt like a complete failure.

I thought I knew what addiction was at the time. I relied on what my drug handbook said about an addict being someone who becomes physically dependent on the substance. I felt if that was what it took for me to get through life, I would be OK. The drug handbook left out the part that I would build up a tolerance to the substances I used and that I would require larger amounts, not just to feel high, but to just feel normal. The handbook omitted that when the pills and alcohol were taken away from me that I would lie, steal, cheat and do just about <u>anything</u> to get what I thought I needed.

It was at about this point in my life when the doctor stopped giving me the pain meds. I was hiding how much I drank at this time and my double life began. On the outside, I was working full-time as a nurse. I was happily married and living in a new home in the town I grew up in. While able to check all of these items off my life's "to do list," on the inside I was insecure, lonely and full of fear. That's where the pills and alcohol came in because they helped me survive.

Close to the top of my life's "to do list" was to be a Mom, which came true as well. I was blessed with a healthy, precious son. Somehow, I was able to stop drinking and using drugs throughout most of my pregnancy. When I delivered him by C-section, however, I was given Tylox for pain and I was off and running again. Even as perfect as my son was, he did not fill that huge, black hole inside of me, so my double life continued full steam ahead.

At this time, I was recruited back to the hospital I had first worked in after nursing school. I was given a new job, which was to help them develop a new Home Health Agency. Although I knew in my gut that I was not right for this job, I took it anyway because of how impressive I thought it made me look. I wanted my parents to be proud of me; the nurse who took so long to get through school but now was a head of a department in our home town hospital.

The next year was a blur. My life became pretty much about survival, which meant find the pills I needed, and hide using them, all the while pretending to be happy. As you might guess, things did not turn out well. I had begun forging prescriptions, a pharmacist caught me and I was turned in to my boss.

An intervention was done by my boss, a nurse from a treatment facility and another pharmacist. I was gently and kindly confronted about the things I had done. At first, I denied what I had done, but then I broke down, admitting everything. It was like a huge weight had been lifted from me. Now the darkest secret of my life was out. I thought I was insane, and I was, but it was also the first time I was told that I was an alcoholic/addict and that there was help for me.

I was taken immediately into treatment. I was being cared for while my outside life crumbled. My parents were left to face the gossip that goes along with a small town nurse stealing drugs and drinking. Going to inpatient treatment also meant leaving my husband with a fifteen month-old child to care for while beginning to sort through all the wreckage I had caused.

No one had known about my double life. My family was in shock. My parents took care of our son, while my husband continued to work and I began the recovery process. I was in treatment for a total of four months, three of which were in a special program for health care professionals. It was during this time that I began to learn to deal with life on life's terms without any mood-altering substances and my family began to heal as well.

Immediately after my four months in treatment, and with my mother's help, I was able to find a job in home health nursing. My manager and I set up a contract at the time to meet weekly and to also have random drug screens done. This was all done on the advice of the treatment facility which I had been in because there were no monitoring programs for nurses in my state at the time. As the AA fellowship is strong in my community that is where I started. So I jumped with both feet into my 12 step program and got a sponsor. I began living life now drug and alcohol-free.

At nine months sober, I went before the Board of Nursing. Because of the things I had done for my recovery and the support I had, I was put on probation for two years and I did not lose my license. I was required to continue with the drug screens and had to report monthly to the nursing board during the period I was on probation.

At the end of this time, things in my state really began to change. The state decided that all health care professionals who had not been prosecuted in the past for criminal acts like forgery would be charged. This was very difficult for me as I thought I had been moving away from my past and building a good future. I was arrested and charged with felonies for the prescriptions I had forged in the past.

The hospital I worked for at the time was very supportive to the extent that they hired an attorney for me and paid all my legal bills. My employer also allowed me to work during the investigation. The outcome was that I was given two years of probation with the matter expunged from my record upon completion of the probationary period.

The next years were spent living what I consider "the good life." My marriage was back on track, our son was doing well and we were building our future. I continued to be active in AA all through this time, until some things began to change. The first thing that changed was that some of my close AA friends stopped coming to meetings. My sponsor, who I had been very close to, moved away and I began to feel so disconnected from the program. This disconnect led me to think I no longer needed meetings since my friends had gone elsewhere. I had a good job, and my marriage and family were good. I had learned my "lesson," so I just stopped going to meetings.

Fast-forward a year and "the good life" began to change. My Dad who was my very best friend and the babysitter for our son began to get ill. I had a new boss who changed things where I worked. We were in the middle of building a brand-new home, which can be a good thing, but is also a stressful thing. So, here I was with big life changes and no tools to deal with them. I reminded myself that after all I had been through I would NEVER repeat my past.

As my Dad's health began to deteriorate, so did mine, at least on the inside. My life became work, helping my Mom care for my Dad and more work. I became filled with fear of what my life and my son's life would be like without my Dad. I worked many hours to build just the right house and turned my back on the wonderful things in my life, like my family.

One day, I could no longer take it and just wanted a break. I took some of my Dad's narcotics, knowing I was flushing my nine years of sobriety down the drain. I just didn't want to feel for awhile and, well, one day led to two, and I was off and running again. The double life I swore I would NEVER go back to, because I knew better, had returned and this time was worse than it had been nine years prior.

My drug supplier became my Dad's meds at first and then, when that was not enough, I stole from the patients in home health who depended on me and trusted me. I did not forge prescriptions again, as I thought I would not leave a paper trail and would not get caught. This was not the case because, after a period of time, one of the nurses I worked with felt something was up. I was confronted at work and fired for the second time in my life

This time, I knew what I was. I was an alcoholic/addict in full relapse who had allowed chemicals to rule her life again. I had tried stopping before I was caught and had tried everything, except telling someone the truth, but I wasn't able to do that.

When I came home the day I was confronted, I was at a turning point. For the rest of my life I will believe that God took over where I could not. I went straight to see a friend who was a recovering pharmacist and, as soon as he saw me, he knew what had happened. He referred me to an organization that had just opened its doors six days prior. They picked me up and began helping me put the pieces of my broken life back together again.

I had broken the trust of my family, my friends and my co-workers. I had confused and hurt the most precious person in my life - my son. This time I had more to lose; and I lost most of it. But, by the grace of God, things did get better.

The monitoring program I signed up for set up a careful plan of care and I followed it to the letter. This plan required 12 step meetings, therapy and weekly random drug screens, all at my own expense. Before, in my first recovery, all this had been paid for by the hospital I worked for.

It took six months, but I was able to find employment in a doctor's office. Ten days after starting this new job, my Dad died. I was heartbroken, but with the tools of the 12 step program, I was able to walk through this sober.

At nine months sober, I went to court for the felonies I had committed while getting the pills I thought I needed. I was certain I was going to jail. Again, by God's grace, the judge had a daughter with my past. Since the judge did not want me to have a felony on my record, the charges were reduced to petty larceny. I was also spared from the loss of my nursing license due to the monitoring program I was in.

Slowly, my life began to get better and, with the help of so many people, the broken pieces began to be put back together.

I feel the monitoring program that I was in saved my life because it was through their direction and care that I made it through some of the most difficult times in early sobriety.

Sober twelve years at this time, I see the world so differently now. I continue to attend three meetings a week. I now hear the message that I missed my first time in recovery: that it's part of my job to keep coming back to pass along the help that was so freely given to me. I no longer wonder if I can make it sober without taking an active part in my recovery, because I know that I cannot. I know that I relapsed not just because my life had gotten painful, but because I stopped being active in my recovery and had no defense against that first drink or that first pill.

My life has actually been enriched by my relapse. To this very day, I do not take for granted that I am sober. I do not take for granted that I am still married to the love of my life, despite all that I put him through. I do not take for granted that I have a good relationship with my son, who turned out to be kind and loving, despite what I put him through. And I do not take for granted that I am able to practice as a Registered Nurse in my state without restrictions on my license.

I am an alcoholic/addict who was once so hopeless. Now, on most days, I am full of hope.

Seduced Into A False Sense Of Security

My career in nursing began somewhat by accident. Although I became a candy-striper in high school and my mother was a nurse, I really wanted to be an artist. That plan was sidelined in the 1960's, however, when I became pregnant at nineteen and got married.

After my son was born, I was granted custody of my fourteen year-old brother-in-law. Since finances were less than optimal and I did not want to wait tables the rest of my life, when I read about an LPN program which offered night classes, I enrolled. Thankfully, my brother-in-law took over the house-keeping and child care duties so I could get through school.

Within the first week of class, I found "my calling," which was taking care of people. Graduating in 1973, I began work-ing as an LPN and, although it took ten years, I was finally able to return to school for my RN. During that ten year span, my second son was born and I was granted custody of my sister-in-law.

Nursing was exciting and I was always looking for new chal-lenges. Although I spent most of my career within the same hospital system, I moved to different departments every three to five years. Starting out in ICU, I went on to pediatrics, al-cohol rehab, psychiatry and the ER. Whatever area I worked in, I would learn all I could about the specialty. Then, after a while, I would become restless and start looking for a new challenge.

In 1989, I found my true niche when I jumped into the back of an ambulance and cross-trained as a paramedic. At that point, I took my "show on the road." Looking back, it was the best time in my career. It was exciting and mentally challenging. I

237

loved the autonomy, and it fed my first addiction, which was adrenalin.

The set-up for where I wound up was that I was diagnosed with Hepatitis C in 2001. I suspect I had it before then because my liver enzymes had been a little high, but the doctor thought I might be fighting off a virus or something. My second marriage of nine years dissolved that same year when my husband who was impacted by the 9-11 terrorist attack didn't handle it well. One day, he just packed all his stuff and moved out. I still haven't gotten over that.

There had been many instances which exposed me to Hep C at work. Being at the bottom end of a stretcher coming down from a third floor walk-up once, a patient's esophageal varices let loose. The blood caught me on the side of the head and ran down my shirt. It's not like I could strip down in the middle of the highway during the forty-five minute trip to the hospital. Another time, I got stuck under an overturned car when I was responding to a motor vehicle accident. In trying to position the man's head to secure an airway, glass went through my glove and cut into the palm of my hand.

I held off on treatment for Hep C, but in 2005, when my liver enzymes went up, was started on Riboviron and Interferon. The doctor required me to be on Zoloft for two weeks before I even started the Interferon. The Hep C therapy made me really, really sick and I wasn't able to work in medical transport at the time. So, I switched over to working in the emergency room, thinking I could handle the ER fast track for three eight-hour shifts a week. By December, though, I could not work at all anymore.

The black box warning notes that Interferon can cause depression. That's an understatement! No longer able to escape into my work and alone in the house by myself, I became very depressed. I got psychotic overlays with the Interferon and, as bizarre as it sounds, I actually wouldn't answer my phone because I thought the hospital had tapped my line. I believed if I talked on the phone, the hospital would know I wasn't really sick, but just faking it. I wouldn't answer the door either and was just hiding out in my house.

Although I managed to rally a bit and convinced my doctor to let me go back to work in May, that only lasted two weeks. Then I got this horrific back pain and was prescribed Percocet. I had a different reaction to the medication, which I'm finding many opiate abusers have. Instead of being tired when taking it, the Percocet acted as a stimulant. Suddenly, I didn't have to go from the couch to a chair only twelve feet away to catch my breath before making my way to the bathroom. I could take four Percocet and actually get up and vacuum the living room.

At the same time, the gentleman next-door passed away from cancer. His wife didn't know what to do with all the leftover meds and I offered to take them to the hospital to get rid of them for her, even though I wasn't working. I thought, "This will work. I can control it. I can handle this and get back to work by taking the Percocet." The drugs were so seductive!

Before this, I'd never had a problem with drugs or alcohol. Although I smoked some grass back in the 1960s, it was mostly when I was at a party, due to peer pressure. I stopped marijuana when I got pregnant without any trouble. I never liked the taste of alcohol or anything that left me feeling out of control or sleepy. Even though I was prescribed amphetamines for weight control from fifth grade through high school until they were banned, I stopped that, too, without any difficulty.

So, the draw to opiates was all this energy that I did not have when I didn't take them. I told myself, "I will just do it today. I will just take it this one time and I'll be feeling better tomorrow. I won't have to do this again." But I did not feel any better the next day and started abusing it.

Although I wasn't a daily user, that in and of itself lulled me further into a false sense of security. Very quickly, my tolerance went up. In addition to the Percocet I was prescribed, I also had a prescription for Dilaudid, which I dissolved and injected to get a greater effect. So, within about four-and-a-half months, I crashed and burned.

I just wanted to go back to my safe place which was work and was becoming more depressed. I also began hating myself for what I had become. So, while trying to go back to work once again, I became seriously suicidal. I acquired some IV Lopressor, a vial of insulin, an IV set-up and a body bag. I didn't have an exact date that I was going to commit suicide, but I had all the equipment I needed and even wrote farewell letters to my children and grandchildren.

My doctor happened to be the infectious disease specialist at the hospital where I worked. I never told him about any of this because I did not want to appear "weak." I wanted to be his "good patient." I never let on how really depressed I was because I felt I would be causing him problems.

Although still suicidal, towards the end of my Interferon therapy, I was able to return to work. When I was back about a month, God intervened when my nurse manager called me into her office, said I wasn't acting like myself and requested a urine drug screen. After I gave the specimen, I called her up and confessed everything.

240

That confrontation threw me into chaos, but I started talking to the employee assistance program personnel. The counselor there didn't think I needed inpatient treatment because I was not an everyday user, so I agreed to go for outpatient treatment. I was given the number of a woman who helps nurses with addiction and was enrolled in the monitoring program for nurses in my state.

Once I completed two months in an outpatient recovery program and my Interferon treatments ended, I was able to think more clearly. I was allowed to go back to work with no restrictions on my license at that time since I hadn't diverted any medications from work. Still, it was pretty difficult to find a job because the monitoring program required me to inform prospective employers that I am in recovery. So, while interviewers would be impressed with my resume, once I told them about the monitoring program, a glaze would come over their eyes. They would get this "deer-in-the-headlights" look at that point.

When I couldn't get a job as a nurse for the first two years I was in the monitoring program, I started working for a veterinarian, cleaning up for horses at a stable during the night. I also did some neonatal intensive care for foals. At this point in my life, I felt like someone took an eraser and wiped away everything I had ever accomplished.

Finally, I found out that one of the other nurses in the monitoring program had been employed at a facility which allowed her to get the help she needed for her addiction, without being fired. Thinking they might be friendly towards me, I applied there and was able to get a per-diem job as a nurse at a school for kids with cerebral palsy. I wish I could say I look forward to going to work when I get to go in, but I can't.

Since then I have also started teaching adult education at a local college for massage therapy students. For the past two years I have talked to the nursing class at a local college, explaining part of what I've gone through. I tell the students about burnout and addiction and how I set myself up by feeling that the hospital was my family. They are not. The hospital is an institution that has to function to make money.

Even though alcohol was not my problem, I attend Alcoholics Anonymous meetings because Narcotics Anonymous is a younger crowd and AA seems to have more sobriety. I've met some neat people there and learned a lot. I realize I was somewhat self-centered and self-absorbed which I never looked at before. I tend to be over-sensitive and think if somebody's in a bad mood, it's about me. I have been able to work past that and I'm better at handling problems now.

Once the Interferon cleared out of my system, I can't say I could identify with people wanting to drink or use drugs anymore. Watching someone have a glass of wine never bothered me before and doesn't now. If I tell people in my nurse support group that I really don't feel like getting stoned or having a drink, some say I'm in denial. I have looked at that and can honestly say that while I did abuse Percocet and Dilaudid and do truly see myself as an addict, I really do not feel like using.

Before all this happened, I started to realize I was getting a little old to be riding around in a truck, carrying stretchers down flights of stairs, but I would have liked to work my way out of it instead of having it ripped away from me. I keep mourning that loss, trying to put to rest the fact that I won't be a medic anymore. I keep working on that.

Drugs do take everything away from you and living with Hepatitis C is like living with a dragon: you never know when he is coming out. Somehow between the two, the Percocet I abused and the Interferon treatment for Hep C, I feel like I have lost my soul. Others I have spoken with in my situation tell me that they feel the same way

My depression lingers, although I have no suicidal plans. I still feel bad about myself and obviously had self-esteem issues before. I had hoped the nurse support group would help me with that. There must be a way for us to talk about how bad we feel, so I plan to work towards building self-esteem for myself and the nurses in my support group.

I feel lucky that I am able to teach adult education with an associate's degree because I am one of those instructors who can get students really excited about learning, even if it is a class most take begrudgingly, like Advanced Coronary Life Support. I would just love to teach nursing school and had planned on going back to school before all this happened. I was going to get a second mortgage to do that, but I used everything I had, first when I was out on disability due to the Interferon, and then when I was unable to find work. While I didn't actually lose my house, a friend of mine bought it and lets me rent half of it.

The gift my Higher Power gave me when I had no job at all was that I was able to fulfill my life-long dream of going to Africa to work in a clinic. Through a friend, I ran into a nun and was able to go to Africa to work in a clinic with her for three weeks.

In the future, I want to network with other nurses who have Hepatitis C and would like to help others realize the potential dangers of the treatment, especially if they're already somewhat depressed. I hope that there is much more research into the possible link I have read about between drug-abuse and Interferon therapy.

When I complete the monitoring program, I'll be sixty-two. I don't look at getting out after five years of monitoring as my release. For over three years now, I've been in recovery, remaining active in AA and speaking at meetings.

Even if I don't really want to (and I often don't want to) I work and do all the things I'm expected to do every day. I use the principle of "One Day at a Time," often feeling like a very tired robot, trying to put a positive spin on everything. It gets exhausting trying to keep up appearances, though, so this is the true me I have shown you, not the one I let most people see.

As nurses we know about drugs, and that puts us at a disadvantage because we can easily be seduced into a false sense of security. Protecting ourselves, giving ourselves time to recuperate when hurt or exhausted, is important. Being especially careful and cautious regarding pain medications is a necessity for us as this was the starting point for many nurses.

Nursing is a wonderful profession, but it is not who we are or our entire life. We are whole human beings, on our own, aside from being nurses. These are the things I wish I had not only learned, but understood, when I started out.

A Miracle Happened In My Life

At twelve years old, I had my first drink. I experimented with some marijuana and different things at that time as well. My road to recovery was difficult, as it is for most addicts and alcoholics. I have found most of our stories are very similar and mine is probably no different in that respect.

The first time I got drunk was at a wedding at the age of thirteen. I share this because what happened that day was obviously not a sufficient event for me never to drink again.

One of my best friends and I were in her sister's wedding party. At the reception, we were allowed to have champagne with the adults. It was December and there were some bowl games on television. Everyone was in a festive mood at the time. I grabbed a hold of the champagne and I remember that I liked the way it made me feel tremendously.

So, I had a bottle-and-a-half of champagne and I became extremely drunk. My tuxedo was hanging out and someone suggested I be taken out for a drive to sober up. There was an older, married man with children who agreed to do that.

At the time, I was blacking out, which was a concept I did not quite understand back then, although I certainly understand it very well today. When I finally woke up, I found myself on a dirt road, being molested.

The next day, although I knew what had happened, I didn't realize the full implications of it. I drank the very next weekend and I was just getting started.

Maybe I had a reason to drink and use drugs at that point, even a lot of alcohol and drugs, but I used that event and subsequent events with that same person as an excuse. I didn't understand what was going on exactly as a thirteen year old because you think you're an adult and understand everything. I did not know for many years how much of an impact this highly inappropriate and completely illegal situation had on me, but I used that event to fuel my alcoholism and drug addiction because I was angry and confused.

I drank throughout high school and in college I began to experiment with drugs, which caused various problems. I had one of those families that would bail me out, though I was never arrested in the early years. I was able to sort of meander through life with no real purpose except to have a good time.

When I was twenty-six years old, I went to nursing school. I tried really hard to do the very best I could in nursing school and finished with a 3.4 grade point average, graduating with honors. I wanted to become a CRNA because I met someone who was a nurse anesthetist. Admittedly, I also wanted to make big bucks and be somewhat prestigious. I thought doing that would make me whole, just like a certain relationship would make me whole or make me whatever I was supposed to be. I thought if I had this certain career, it would make me attractive. That would make me OK with life. That's one of the main reasons I became a nurse, although later on that would all implode upon itself.

In nursing school I was a weekend warrior. I managed to do very well throughout the week and would go out with friends and have a good time on weekends. The pattern throughout my life had always been that whenever I would start drinking, I would binge drink. I didn't know what was going to happen, where I was going to end up or who was going to have to take care of me. Once I started drinking, I didn't know what my behavior would be.

Oftentimes I would wake up very remorseful and ashamed of what had happened and who it had happened with, if I was lucky enough to remember at all. Generally, I could piece things together but even today I sometimes get those blurbs of "Oh my God, that happened that night." If I truly knew everything that did happen, I don't know if I could handle it all at once, so I think that is a protection from God. I'm able to deal with the memories at the time God lets me see and remember them.

Throughout nursing school, I was really just maintaining my drinking. I had no idea that I was an alcoholic, even though during that time I got a DUI. I was able to get an attorney and "get out" of that DUI charge because I was very close to the legal limit. But even with all that trouble, I still didn't think I had a problem with alcohol or drugs.

Continuing on my journey, I went to work in a hospital. In looking back, I think I never really cared about what I was doing, only about achieving the means to the end that I wanted. In other words, I needed to get ICU experience so that I could become a CRNA, but I wasn't thinking about what I could do for these patients, or this hospital, or the people around me. It was all me, me, me.

It was all about how I could get what I wanted with the least effort possible. Granted, as every nurse knows, going to nursing school is no easy feat; but the mindset wasn't there for me to truly be a nurse for the reason most nurses choose to become a nurse. I know my intent was certainly not pure or even probably fifty percent pure; I wanted what I wanted.

I worked in home health and ICU and did a couple of different things as a nurse which were good experiences for me. I was the type, however, who would work somewhere for a little while and then miss a few days of work due to my alcoholism. At this time, I wasn't diverting from the facilities yet. I was able to get what I needed and did not even think about diverting because I was not really taking prescription medication at this point. Or, if I did ever think about diverting, I would become afraid that I was going to get caught if I did that, so I got what I needed elsewhere.

In the beginning of my career, my resume was very patchy because I would go somewhere and be scared I was going to have a drug test. So, I would give my notice and go somewhere else. The beauty of being a nurse addict is that we can go anywhere with a sketchy resume and get a job because we're in high demand, or so it seems.

Many times I was probably not totally honest about where I had worked or for how long. I listed only the places where I had been for at least a year. I was micromanaging life at this level to cover up something that I was just becoming aware of. I didn't understand this until many years later. It's a lot of work to live in addiction and to cover up things with the plans, schemes and designs that I had to in order to keep up what I felt were good appearances on the outside with family, friends, jobs and relationships.

I could never really form a true partnership or friendship with another person because I usually pissed them off or took everything I could from them. Then they often didn't want anything to do with me. I was told later on that my behavior was very erratic. I didn't understand that for awhile and just thought how could they be such jerks to stop being my friend?

Finally, I did go to anesthesia school, which is what I had set out to do originally. I was no stranger to prescription pain and sleep medication when I entered school. Someone had shown me a few years previously that I could go to these websites and order whatever I wanted. Sure enough, I grabbed a credit card, placed an order and there it was at my front door: Lortab, Xanax, or whatever. I charged up a lot of debt to feed my addiction this way.

I knew I had a problem and kept telling myself that I had to quit. I would get close friends who knew my habits, who were the only friends I had left, to help me try to come off the medications. But I could not stop because if I went through the withdrawal process, I didn't have a solution. I didn't have an answer or a solution to why I kept going back to using and drinking.

One day, almost two years into anesthesia school, I was in the OR and had a very stressful day. The surgeon had nicked a patient's artery and a simple outpatient procedure had suddenly become a huge deal, with blood going everywhere. I was calling for backup and putting in a central line, which I'd done a few times before as a senior.

Although the patient ultimately did well, it was very stressful for me. For some reason, when I got relieved after that case to go to the bathroom, I had all this Versed, fentanyl, and other stuff that anesthetists keep in their pockets. I was just stressed at the time and remember thinking that diabetics are able to give themselves shots, so "why not me?"

Without even another thought, I took the syringe with the leftover fentanyl and injected it intramuscularly in my butt. I was scared about what would happen but I also knew I had a tolerance from the drugs I had been taking. Within five or ten minutes, I started to feel better than I had ever felt in my life. I knew I had just stumbled onto something extraordinary in my world of addiction and alcoholism. I felt so relaxed that it was really scary but, at the time, I didn't think about that.

That wonderful justification and rationalization that I can do this because it was just going to be wasted medication set in. So, I continued to do it and, for about a month, I was just doing intramuscular injections.

I still remember the day I switched to intravenous use, though, and thinking that I needed to use a very tiny needle, like an insulin syringe. I was so scared because I had never done this before. I was in the bathroom at work and stuck that little bitty needle into my vein. The effect of the fentanyl was magnified even more at that point and I was really off to the races.

Within three or four months, I was just a basket case. I felt like my mind was going to explode. I could not keep up with the deception and was always scrambling to see if my records were right; if I was charting too much or too little. I always wondered if this was the day I was going to get caught. I made all these crazy rules as alcoholics and addicts do, like I was not going to take the drug out of the facility because that was wrong. It was OK for me to steal it from patients while I was at work, though.

At home at night, I would go through horrible withdrawals, so I'd drink to fight that off. A cycle had set in, so, once again, it was time for me to tuck and run. Here I am, about a month before completing anesthesia school, and I was absolutely a basket case, thinking I am going to get caught. I asked to be transferred somewhere else and all the questions started about why I wanted to leave to go elsewhere. If I could just get some psychological counseling, I could figure out what was going on and stop!

Once placed in a new facility, they were onto me very quickly. I was intervened upon within a couple weeks and asked to submit to a series of drug tests. That was my bottom. I had a moment of clarity which was literally four days before school was out. I remember talking to my dean on the phone, having the feeling that, finally, the jig was up. I had nothing left to hide, so I told her I was terribly addicted to fentanyl and that I needed help.

Off to treatment I went and, for the first time in a long while, I had a little bit of hope. My bottom was sufficient enough that I began to think anything would be better than the way I was living. Granted, there was a lot of fear involved and I wanted to keep my career. I also wanted to graduate but, at the same time, I was desperately miserable in my addiction. I was sick and tired of living the way that my addiction made me live for so long.

After a couple weeks of going through withdrawal in the treatment facility, my mind started to come back. I began to really have this feeling of hope that I could actually go for days and weeks without putting a mind changing substance in my body. That was amazing to me because it had never happened to me before. After I had a month without a substance or a drink, I was amazed that I had been able to go for a month without using after fifteen years of non-stop use. I had not yet realized I had nothing to do with it, but once I started wrapping my brain around that idea, I began to really think that something had shifted in me. Life was going to be better.

It was a real struggle to attempt to finish school but I received a lot of help from the American Association of Nurse Anesthetists' Peer Assistance Committee. A lot of people were really trying to fight for me. At the time, I lived in a disciplinary state, which meant that they imposed direct action on my nursing license. It all ended up in a legal battle that lasted three years which required my family and me to make some big decisions because my addiction would be made public. The matter was in the newspapers but I was told that was just part of the legal process.

Ultimately, I was suspended from school because direct action was being taken on my license. I couldn't be in the classroom setting with an encumbered license, even though the Board of Nursing said I could go back to school. It was just a mess. I never knew situations like this existed before.

Although I really don't know for sure, I think the dean may have felt her hands were tied. Certainly there was no love lost between the program director and myself and rightfully so as I look back on it, because I had probably worn her out with my addictive behavior. Relationships can be damaged so badly that people just do not want to help you. It took me a long time to understand and accept that.

So, I got out of treatment, got a sponsor and worked the 12 steps of Alcoholics Anonymous. At that point, my life began to change. My first sponsor was a lady because I didn't trust men. She was very kind, but when we got to steps four and five and I did my fear inventory, she said, "You are going to have to get a man to be your sponsor now."

To this day, I am so grateful she did that because I have many men who are my friends today whom I trust. There is a mutual respect for who they are and who I am. It was tremendous to be able to do that. So I was able to go through the steps with a man who taught me how to be a friend to another man, something I never thought I could do. That was one of the many fears in my fear inventory.

As I went through the Big Book with my sponsor, he taught me how to pray following the directions that are laid out in the book. When it said to make a decision in step three and to pray, we prayed. We got on our knees together and took the third step prayer. We moved through the inventory and read the book together, every word in the first 164 pages, and I was willing to do what he told me to do. I was willing to take that action.

I think my life really changed when I got the chance to make amends and looked at steps eight and nine for the first time. I went to old places, saw people from the past and put myself out there, saying, "I'm an alcoholic. I owe you this" or "I did something wrong and I am here to make it right." I was extremely afraid to do that whether it was Walmart or some of these places I'd stolen from when I was younger and drunk, or even when I was not drunk. Whatever the case was, I learned that I had lived with all that "stuff" and that the shame just fed my alcoholism. It was amazing to walk through that fear.

The way to release it was to go clean up my side of the street. To this day, I still work on that. It will be a lifelong process to clean up my side of the street however the program gives me the tools to be able to do it.

Not all of my amends were met with people saying, "Good for you." Some of those old relationships were so damaged, torn and tormented, that I didn't even get so much as a "Hey. Glad you got your life together." In one of those situations where I didn't realize how badly I hurt someone, I got no word back at all. I tried a couple times until finally she got word through to a mutual friend who told me to leave her alone.

I remember initially thinking, "I am sober. What is going on here?" My sponsor, though, told me I'd made my attempt and to leave it alone. He explained that I'm not always going to get the response that I want, the way that I want it. Overwhelmingly, though, the responses to the amends I've made have been tremendous.

I have been fortunate to be able to work with some other guys in the program by sponsoring them. I've been able to see how this amends process works through them as well as myself.

Now I am working through the steps again, four-and-a-half years later, with another sponsor because my first sponsor had moved away. I felt that I needed to revamp my program this last year and I am working on steps eight and nine again right now. There are some things I need to look at that I didn't see the first time around.

This program has given me more than I could ever ask for. It truly is a design for living that has given me a relationship with a Higher Power and the ability to be among other people in the world without being constantly consumed with fear. It has certainly allowed me to do so without putting alcohol in my body or putting a needle in my arm every day. That is an absolute miracle.

Sometimes I forget that, though; that it's not me running the show. It's not because I'm so smart and so good, or that I've read everything and studied hard and taken all the notes and learned it. It's all because a miracle happened in my life.

Today, I try to help other recovering nurses, especially student nurses. I learned in my situation that there were a lot of policy issues that needed a lot of work, specifically around the situation with recovering nurses. As I learned about the policy issues that needed to be changed, I began to learn that writing about them and researching them was probably the best way for me to get a message out to people who could make a difference. It also helped me to work through a lot of my own anger, guilt, fear and shame. It was another inventory process to be able to write about changing the future for another nurse and to hopefully help someone else because of my experience.

Today it's like I'm a kid all over again. I'm thirty-nine years old, nearly five years sober and feel like I'm sixteen. I will be completing a PhD in nursing in a couple of months. Recovery and God have been so good to me.

I have more energy than I have ever had in my life. Though I never used to work out before, I exercise all the time now. It just feels so good to take care of myself instead of just destroying my body with drugs and alcohol. Every single day is an adventure. Though some days may seem completely awful, there is a solution. That's the beauty of it all!

Prayed For The Willingness To Be Willing

There was this very small but persistent voice inside me that said, "Don't cross that line. You'll get caught." I remember to this very day how difficult that struggle was with the opposite thought, almost a command, saying, "You need to get this. You don't need to go back to the doctor. You have been ordered this and you're a nurse so you can write the prescription yourself."

I'd only been a nurse for a few short years in the 1970s and felt I "knew enough" being a nurse. I thought that once I was prescribed a medication by a doctor, there was really no need for any reevaluation by a middleman, which I saw as an unnecessary step. Since prescription pads were as readily available on every hospital unit as scratch paper, the implement was more than accessible. I downplayed the importance, as well as the accuracy, of the term "forgery" and tried to deny the illegality of what I was tempted to do.

Looking back, I see I was not only supremely blessed, but extremely lucky to have had that voice that chanted, "Don't. You'll regret it." While I thank heaven that I listened to the voice of caution, for many years I forgot about that struggle between the temptation of a thrifty short-cut and the boundaries defining my scope of practice.

I was set-up from birth to have an addictive lifestyle. It was, however, a preordained path, more like a rut in life, that I did not have to go down very far or long before being turned on to recovery. This is not at all to my credit. Generations before me of fraternal and maternal grandparents had serious issues with alcohol, so I saw clearly and early-on that theirs was a life that was not at all what I wanted.

While I would not label my fraternal grandmother technically an alcoholic, every Thanksgiving after over a dozen grandchildren and a score of aunts and uncles were served the feast to end all feasts, she would "relax" with a bottle of Tawny Port. Everyone present knew very well from the holidays past that once she had even one sip, she was off to the races. Her face would go crimson, all of a sudden. She would get loud, a bit rambunctious, and say things that would be extremely hurtful to some of her guests, especially the daughter-in-laws. I remember that to this day and know that I certainly have that same genetic predisposition.

My father was an alcoholic who, to my knowledge, never entered recovery, even though in his later years, before he died, he did not drink as much. When I was young, though, he was a very violent, nasty drunk. He did not drink in the home, but would drink after work, in the bar with his buddies in the construction trade. That was a very acceptable form of commiserating with coworkers back then and still seems to be a part of that industry even today.

Both of my grandfathers were very heavy drinkers and at least one customarily beat his wife. While violence may not be as closely associated with genetics as addiction, I did witness my own mother being physically abused by my father as early as age four. It always occurred when he was drunk and certainly had a negative impact on me.

My mother's response to my father's drinking and abusiveness, both physical and emotional, was to overeat and smoke cigarettes. I vividly recall that my very first addiction started rather innocuously by binging on foods high in sweets, carbs and fats as a teenager.

Although I went on to steal cigarettes from my mother as a teen, I never felt the need to smoke regularly until after I had graduated from nursing school. However, once I began working as a registered nurse, I had a great need to self-medicate the extreme deluge of stress I encountered on the job as a new grad, that I began smoking regularly. This was back at a time when there were none of the prohibitions against smoking in hospital cafeterias or coffee shops which exist today. So, I began smoking regularly with my colleagues on coffee breaks and at mealtimes.

I remember I bummed a cigarette from one of the many nurses who smoked back then on the medical floor I worked on. Actually, I bought my very first pack of cigarettes a mere day or so later in the hospital coffee shop because I felt so lousy borrowing cigarettes from my coworker. I pretty much became a pack-a-day smoker at that point; literally overnight.

Since I had an eating disorder like my mother, one of my reasons for starting to smoke was that it helped me curtail my eating. Like every addict, I never saw what was coming next because I then wound up with two uncontrollable facets in my life: compulsive overeating and nicotine addiction.

In hindsight I can also see that during this same period I had already begun to travel down the road of problematic alcohol use. While I had sworn to myself that I would never have an alcohol problem like my Dad, before I graduated nursing school I had lost a day from work due to the overconsumption of scotch. Since I was self-supporting through my own contributions and no one else's at the time, this was a huge deal as no show at my job equated to no pay.

So, I figured that the best way to eliminate that type of problematic behavior was to just stop drinking scotch. So at that point, I switched to screwdrivers and shortly thereafter, when screwdrivers became a problem, I eliminated screwdrivers and switched to sombreros. When sombreros became a habitual fiasco, they were ruled out too, and I switched to wine. From wine, I went to wine spritzers.

It wasn't until years later, when I achieved abstinence from in Overeaters Anonymous, that I totally stopped using alcohol. That just became a part of my recovery program. It was not until about six months after what has proved to be my last drink in 1982, however, that I was assaulted with an almost irresistible craving for alcohol. I did not want a drink or even a few. What I wanted, almost needed, was a half-gallon; a big sledge hammer to obliterate all feelings, permanently.

So, at that time it became painfully obvious to me that I had unknowingly crossed over that invisible line into alcoholism without ever having more of an aftermath than most people consider their customary "right of passage" from adolescence into adulthood. At the time, I admitted to myself and my closest of confidantes that I certainly fit one of the many definitions of an alcoholic because surely I had become someone who couldn't predict with reasonable certainty what would happen if they picked up a drink again.

The Twelve Steps and Twelve Traditions of Overeaters Anonymous, which I firmly believe in along with all of the suggestions of Alcoholics Anonymous, describe the recovery process as an ongoing refinement of character. In pursuit of that objective, I started to become increasingly troubled by my cigarette smoking. It took another solid year for me to feel comfortable enough in my recovery from overeating and alcohol to turn my attention towards quitting cigarettes.

259

In 1984, I started praying for the "willingness to be willing" to quit smoking. Here I was, in a 12 step program for my over-eating which included abstinence from all alcohol, and I just started praying for the "willingness to be willing" to stop smoking. I knew I was not even close to being willing to quit at that point. In fact, I was really not even close to a state of willingness to even <u>be</u> willing to stop, yet I knew that I desperately needed the basic rudiments of willingness in order to succeed in quitting permanently.

So I prayed, at first very reluctantly and gingerly, not at all wholeheartedly or in earnest at the time. I knew from my past experience letting go of excess food and all alcohol that any "willingness to be willing" would only come after I had suffered enough pain. I figured that pain would probably come from burning a certain quota of clothing I truly loved or other items I had come to treasure. I knew a certain amount of pain would be absolutely necessary before I would possess true willingness anywhere near the dimension I needed in order to quit smoking entirely. Yes, some things burned.

Months later, I found myself at the brink of a miracle; a point where I had never been in all the years I had smoked. The window to release was opened ever so slightly when I found one morning that I had not smoked for twelve hours. By this point, quitting had become so fear provoking and panic inducing that I was up to three packs per day for several months. I hadn't been feeling well physically but that had never stopped me or even prompted me to cut down before. To illustrate just how powerful my nicotine addiction was, although I am ashamed to admit it, I was incapable of even cutting down my consumption in response to being pregnant with either of my children.

Here I was, twelve very long hours without even a drag, and I realized at that very juncture that, whether I liked it or not, at some point, I would be separated from my beloved cigarettes. I could either have some say in the timing of that departure from my security blanket of smoking, if I took this twelve hour opportunity and ran with it; or, at some other point, not at all of my choosing, the matter would be decided for me. My mother had not yet been diagnosed with lung cancer, which she would later die from, but I knew the risk smoking was to my health and the likely scenarios continued smoking would lead to.

Then it dawned on me that the twelve hours free of nicotine I was experiencing at that moment, and have continued to experience every moment since that October day in 1984, could be managed with the simple recognition and acceptance that I truly was, and remain, only one puff away from no less than three packs a day. It was that awareness which greatly helped me get through the first six months of a tortuous withdrawal process, which included severe malaise, anxiety and depression. Using all the tools in the arsenal I had established in OA, I was able to quit smoking, maintain my abstinence from compulsive overeating and alcohol, and maintain my goal weight.

Decades later, when I heard a speaker mention the temptation she once had as a nurse to forge a prescription that she, too, resisted, I recalled my own past thoughts of forging a prescription. I marveled then, as I do now, at just how lucky she and I both were; yet became curious about how many nurses succumb to such a thought.

While the drugs that proved problematic for me were food, nicotine and alcohol, I could have very easily fallen into a dependency upon prescription and illicit substances. That such a fate was not to become part of my story is, once again, not to my credit, but I do know that the temptation to forge a prescription was sparked by the appetite suppressant I was legitimately prescribed in the 1970s. Manipulating the dose from the very start, I was a time bomb that was fortunately defused by the repeated chants from the voice of caution. The bomb was totally disarmed by my entry into OA and other fellowships such as AA and Adult Children of Alcoholics.

Had lighting the fuse of forgery been part of my story, I have no doubt that life as I knew it would have ceased. There were no alternative to discipline programs back then. I would have lost a whole lot more than my license as my entire identity and self-worth was all wrapped up in being a nurse back then.

While being a nurse still defines much of who I am and what I do, I have learned, by necessity, to identify myself first as a recovering compulsive overeater, former smoker and alcoholic in recovery. Very gratefully, I never had to traverse through the later stages of those addictive disorders which actually manifested themselves in so many of my family members.

While I count my lucky stars every single day that I did not have to go down the road that many nurses have gone down, I understand completely how nurses and others are seduced by mood-altering substances and behaviors.

There is a most definite stigma which can be cut with a knife regarding having a chemical dependency if you are a nurse. It saddens me deeply to read or hear the profoundly demeaning comments that are made about nurses who have diverted or forged prescriptions which are frequently made by those within and outside of nursing. Such remarks would never be tolerated if they were written or said about any other group. I've heard more compassionate commentary uttered about terrorists than nurses with addiction.

Addiction is a disease; never a choice. While there may be one momentary decision which could qualify as a volitional act to use, the fact is that for many nurses that first decision to use is the last time that their free-will is totally functional.

The only remedy for me and many others I have met in recovery is something intangible which comes from outside of us. Whatever that "something" is, it just appears to mingle with our very feeblest attempt to stop. At least, that was my impression when I was not capable of any more than a half-hearted willingness to achieve abstinence.

I hope that the future holds as much sensitivity and compassion for nurses with addictive disorders as most of us have learned, either by choice or through legal statute, to grant to minorities and culturally diverse groups. At the very least, we need to extend sensitivity to those who are active in their addiction as well as those who are in recovery or susceptible to becoming addicted. Surely, no one preselects their genetic make-up in the hopes of becoming addicted; nor does anyone choose addiction as a life path or occupational track.

Through Doing It My Way

Between the age of three and twelve, I was sexually abused by an uncle. Although I don't blame my alcoholism on that, it certainly set the stage for having feelings to drink over, like my feelings of self-hatred, dirtiness, feeling less than and alone.

My parents never knew that I was abused because I never told them. Almost every weekend, they brought my sister and I over to my uncle's house where he had free reign with us. My aunt was deaf and she left for work each morning at two a.m. to do the baking for a near-by restaurant. There was no phone at my uncle's house, so I could not simply call my parents. I was really a captive audience.

During the time I was abused, I started stuttering very badly. When the abuse stopped, the stuttering stopped. It was like I was holding all this stuff in; not even willing to let words come out of my mouth.

Looking back, my mother used to give my sister and I castor oil when we were young for the frequent constipation we had. Now I see that the holding in of stool, as well as the holding in of everything else inside me, was related to the sexual abuse.

I come from a very poor family. We lived in a house in the city and did not even have a shower or a tub. Our toilet was actually in a closet.

Being a very quiet, shy kid, I wasn't part of any group and really had no peers. After sixth grade, all the children in my class were sent on to seventh grade in one school while I was sent to another school in the area. When I told one of my classmates that I was the only one going on to seventh grade in the other school, I remember her looking me straight in the eye, saying, "That's alright. You're not well liked anyway."

The only way I had to feel good about myself when I was young was to study. I felt if I got all A's on my report card I must be a good person. So, that was my life: studying and getting good grades. Even today at sixty-three years of age I still enjoy studying. I am very glad I was able to channel all that negative energy into something positive to get me to where I am today.

When I was fifteen, I met my husband. I remember that day well because my dog had gotten away from me. I was chasing my dog up the street with my hair in rollers and a hairnet over them at the time. I was really a bad sight and did not realize there was a guy going down the other side of the street. He saw me and wanted to meet me.

I found out later that he had asked around the neighborhood until he found somebody who knew me, so he could be properly introduced. Looking back, had he done it any other way, it would have been unacceptable to me because I just couldn't tolerate any type of forwardness due to the sexual abuse.

We dated and made some pretty mature decisions for our age. After high school, I went to nursing school on a Monday and he went into the army that same week on Friday. We both did our three years, me in school and he in the service, so we wouldn't be bothering each other. Three years later, we planned our wedding for the following May.

Growing up, there wasn't any alcohol in my house. I remember my first drink like it was yesterday. I was a goody-two-shoes who played by the rules, so I didn't have that first drink until I was twenty-one years old. It was a couple weeks after my twenty-first birthday, when I went to a restaurant with two of the girls from nursing school. I thought to myself, "Oh. I can have a drink now because I'm twenty-one."

So, I had one drink, a daiquiri, and I can tell you an alcoholic was born that night. The obsession began from that very first drink. I wanted to know when I could have another drink. The thought of going into a bar wasn't even on my radar screen but I'd look forward to the next wedding or another event so I could have a drink.

I remember as a student in my psychiatric rotation, we had to go to an Alcoholics Anonymous meeting to see what it was like. I heard the story of a woman there who was about fifty years-old. She said she didn't drink during the day, but every single night when she came home she had to drink. At the time, I just thought she was such a poor thing to be that addicted and tied down. Well, fast forward to twenty-two years later and that was me.

After we got married, since it was my place now, I could have alcohol in the house. My drinking started off very slowly which is a pretty typical story from what I've read about the alcoholic who does not use any drugs. It usually takes about twenty years to hit bottom in cases like that and that was certainly true of me. My drinking increased very slowly over a long period of time.

When I had been married a little over a year, I had my first blackout. We had moved to another town and my husband was going to join the Veterans of Foreign Wars since he was a Viet Nam veteran. So, we went to the VFW hall one Saturday night. All the guys there wanted to buy me a drink to be hospitable since my husband was a new member. I lost count at fourteen drinks.

At that time in our marriage, I would strip the bed every Saturday morning and then on Saturday night my husband and I would make the bed together. When I got up Sunday morning after that first night at the VFW hall, I asked my husband who had made the bed the night before. He said, "We did. Don't you remember?" But I couldn't even remember coming home that night.

To this day, if anybody ever says, "Don't you remember?" it really is like a kick in the stomach to me because there were a lot of times that I didn't remember. In fact, at the end of my drinking, I blacked out every single night.

A couple years into the marriage, I had my son which really escalated my drinking. As I look back now, I wasn't really ready to have a child even though I was twenty-four at the time. I didn't feel I had the mother genes or the instincts of a mother.

It was very difficult for me to care for my son even though I was an obstetrical nurse who also taught obstetrics at that time. Although I could teach mothers how to take care of their babies, I had a really hard time doing it myself. Since my husband worked very long hours as an oil burner repair man, this meant that I spent a lot of time alone with my son. I really didn't want to be left alone with my son because I was afraid but I was basically filling the role of both mother and father since when my husband was home he was usually sleeping.

So I would drink when my son went down for a nap or when he went to bed at night. I apparently hid my drinking well from my son because when I told him I was going into treatment for alcohol when he was seventeen years old, he didn't believe me. He didn't even know that I drank alcohol.

The only one who knew about my drinking was my husband. Even the nurse I had worked with and known since ninth grade didn't know that I drank. I never drank at work, before work or at lunch, but at the end of the work day, when I got home at five o'clock, nothing would stop me.

There were no DWIs because I didn't drink and drive. I played by the rules, with that big "R" of responsibility on my chest. I didn't drink in bars, so I didn't wake up in any unfamiliar places. I drank at home, at first mixing my drinks, shaking the liquids up, straining them into a nice glass and all of that. By the bitter end, I was drinking Southern Comfort straight out of the bottle as soon as I got home from work.

Many of my drinking experiences were very embarrassing rather than being filled with legal problems. My son was friends with the minister's son as a child and went to stay overnight at the minister's house when he was around twelve. I was to pick him up the next morning, so after my son left the house, I was all set to drink. When I heard the back door open around eight o'clock and saw my son with the minister's wife and her son, I was there on the couch, already one-half to three-quarters sloshed, wearing a nightshirt that said, "I'm in heat."

While that slogan really referred to my husband's heating business, it was quite embarrassing. Years later, when I told that story to someone who wasn't an alcoholic, pointing out how embarrassed I was, her response was, "Can you imagine how your son felt?" Until then, I had never even thought about that because everything was all about me back then.

When my son was fourteen, he went to the mall with one of his friends one Saturday. The other boy's mother was going to pick them up. My son was to stay overnight and I was to pick him up the next morning. I started drinking but around eight o'clock that night I got a phone call from the security guard at the mall. I was informed that my son was found on the rooftop of the mall with his friend. They wanted me to come to pick up my son at the security office.

My husband was home that night, so he drove us to the mall where I told him that I'd just sit in the car and wait for them. My husband got out of the car and said, "Yeah, because you're drunk, that's why." There were very few times in my twenty-one years of drinking that my husband ever commented about my drinking. He was a great enabler and I certainly took advantage of that.

Since our family was very closed mouthed all around, I didn't know that my sister was an alcoholic until she was about nine or ten years sober. Around 1982 when our mother died, I told my sister I had a problem with drinking and couldn't stop. I followed my admission of a problem up by saying, "Now that you know, I'll be able to stop because since you know, I'll be accountable." Her response was, "Would it be the same thing if you had a heart attack? You would be OK and never have another heart attack just because I knew?" That hit me right between the eyes because she put it on a level that I understood. It still didn't stop me from drinking, however.

When we moved into a brand new house we had built from scratch in 1986, I felt like I had finally arrived. It had two full baths, a circular driveway, a pool and a deck. About three weeks later, after one of the worst hangovers I had ever had in my life, I called my sister who lived over a thousand miles away. At the time she had over sixteen years in recovery at the time.

For five years, I had been counseling employees as an Employee Assistance Program case manager. Even though I was well aware of what treatment programs were available, I asked my sister to give me a referral to treatment. When she found an outpatient treatment program for me, I went to work that day and got an appointment for an evaluation that coming Monday.

After I made that appointment, I went over to get my yearly evaluation from my boss. It is ironic that this was truly one of the lowest points in my life and yet my employee evaluation rating at the time went from "commendable" to "highly commendable." That evaluation reflects the overachiever in me who always overcompensated for what I thought were my inadequacies by really cranking out the work.

After receiving this evaluation, I asked my boss if I could leave work early for a doctor's appointment and went to treatment. I was instructed to go to a meeting every day, get a sponsor and become active in the Alcoholics Anonymous program. Although I thought to myself, "Are they crazy?" I did go to one or two meetings a week and attended weekly individual and group sessions at the program. Of course, I did not lose any time from work and kept right on working because my work was so important to me.

A year-and-a-half after I was in outpatient treatment, I was able to put only six months of sobriety together and was discharged from treatment. Big mistake! Within two months of leaving treatment, I was drinking worse than ever and I went downhill very fast.

For the last six months of my drinking, I bought a small bottle, a pint, on the way home from work every day because each day was going to be my last day drinking. I stopped on the way home from work, bought a bottle of one hundred proof Southern Comfort and would start drinking right out of bottle once I got home, around five o'clock. I'd sneak the alcohol by having it in the other room, every ten or fifteen minutes going to the other room to take a quick swig.

By five-thirty or six o'clock each night, I would be totally plastered. By eight o'clock I would be passed out. I would come to at about one o'clock each morning with my heart pounding out of my chest and my mouth filled with cotton. My stomach would be in my throat. I would lie awake like that until about five a.m. which is when I finally fell asleep, only to wake up an hour later to throw up, take a shower, get dressed, smack a smile on my face and go to work saying, "I'm not going to drink again."

Then, in spite of all that, I would stop on the way home, buy a pint bottle, start drinking right from the bottle as soon as I got home, to black out, pass out, come to, fall asleep at five, wake up at six, throw up, take a shower, get dressed, smack a smile on my face, go to work and repeat that vicious cycle, every single day.

Although I was a very high functioning alcoholic, I was afraid it was going to start interfering with my work. I was afraid that I would have a blackout at work and an employee would call-in saying they would be out sick for awhile and that I wouldn't remember to document it. If that happened, the employee would be fired. Even the fear of being blacked out every night, not knowing if someone from my car pool called to say they weren't going to be in the next day scared me.

271

It got to the point that I just couldn't look at myself. I actually felt lower than a snake at this time because how could I possibly take care of you if I could not take care of myself? I couldn't stand myself anymore because I was living a double life. It was like I was two entirely different people: a professional by day and a drunk by night. I thank God that those two lives never crossed paths.

Once again, I called my sister, told her I just couldn't do it anymore and was afraid I was going to lose my nursing license. I remember her telling me at the time that I was going to have to take that chance. When I knew I was ready to put my nurse's license on the line to get the help I needed, I knew that I was finally ready to recover.

Looking back, it was the fear of being found out that was the worst fear of all. I think that directly related to the fear of being found out when I was a kid being sexually abused. When the abuse first started, I didn't know what it was all about. Then, when old enough to know what it was all about, I didn't tell anybody because then they would say it was my own fault because I let it go on.

When I went to bed the night of April 20th, 1988, it was the first time in a long while I didn't blackout. I remember going to bed that night, saying out loud, "God help me." I didn't say please or get on my knees, but I said out loud, "God help me."

The next morning, I got up, told my husband I couldn't take drinking anymore and that I was going into treatment. He said, "Whatever you think is best." I remember calling my boss that day and told her I wasn't coming in because I was going into treatment for alcohol. She really didn't believe I had a problem until later on, when I told her part of my story.

So I called a small inpatient treatment place for women only. Their clients were predominantly professional women, mostly nurses, and all the counselors were recovering nurses. I told myself if the nurses working there were doing OK, maybe someday I would be OK.

If you were to look at my check register for April 21st, 1988, you would see all the entries I made to pay all the bills for the coming month. Still being that person with the big "R" of responsibility on my chest, I wanted to make sure that everything was in order.

I was able to stay inpatient for thirty days at the time because it was before managed care came about. I went to meetings and had group and individual counseling every day. Even though I was truly exhausted when I left treatment, I went to a meeting the very night I came home and joined an AA group. I continued to go to a meeting every single day.

When my boss asked, "How can I help you?" I said, "Well, there's a meeting up the street that starts at four o'clock. If I could possibly leave work five minutes early at four twenty-five, I could beat the traffic and get half of that meeting in." My boss suggested, "Why don't you leave at four o'clock and get the whole meeting in?"

The flexibility my boss gave me was great and I did what she suggested for awhile. As time went on, I left later than four o'clock but at least I had the option to leave. When it really counted, my boss backed me up, trusted me and didn't question me. I had been truthful with her. I even told her that if I started drinking again she would be able to tell because I would avoid her like the plague, especially in the morning.

From then on, I kept going to AA meetings. I went on to be active as group secretary, booking speakers and went on commitments. I got a sponsor, worked my program like I was supposed to and have not had a drink since April 20th, 1988.

Although I can honestly say that covering up my drinking took more energy than it did for me to get and stay sober, my gambling story isn't so pretty. I have come to find that just because I or anyone else has a solid path of continuous recovery in one addiction does not necessarily mean that is the case with every other addiction.

While the timeline and circumstances surrounding my alcoholism are vivid, my GA recovery is rather blurry. I do know that in 1992, a casino opened in a neighboring state. Before that time, I had occasionally enjoyed going to the local dog track. Although I liked it, I was doing nothing big time as far as gambling.

One night, I remember going to the casino alone after work. I remember telling someone I was just going to see what it was like. I planned on spending about a hundred dollars and when I went, I couldn't even spend the hundred dollars. So I spent forty or fifty dollars gambling that night and came home.

It was not until later on when the casino added the slot machines that I went back. It was a rather social thing to do with friends or people from work. I started going to the quarter slot machine and I can equate it as being very similar to the progression of the alcoholic. I went from the twenty-five cent machines to the fifty cent machines. From there, I progressed to the dollar machines and then went up from there. The frequency of my gambling also increased and I started going without anyone else.

In 1999 or 2000, I felt it was becoming a problem and I was able to quit on my own around January of 2000 or 2001. The eighth day after I quit, however, is quite memorable because I happened to go with a friend to a very special athletic event. It was a Saturday and we had box seats with food and all that went along with having a box seat for this special game.

While I really enjoyed the event, I told my friend afterwards that I didn't want to be alone. At first, we went to a bookstore and had some hot chocolate. Then we went somewhere else and eventually came home.

Today, I can clearly see that I was experiencing withdrawal symptoms from not gambling for eight days straight. I can honestly say that the withdrawal I had from gambling was far worse than any withdrawal symptoms I ever had from alcohol.

I really don't know exactly how long I went without gambling. At one point, I remember having dinner with a friend who asked how I was doing and I admitted that I was gambling inter- mittently again. As she was an Employee Assistance Program professional, she gave me a referral to an outpatient treatment program for gambling.

So in 2002, I went for outpatient treatment for gambling which included individual and group counseling as well as edu- cational sessions. Being a nurse with a master's degree in substance abuse counseling, I acted more like I was the group leader than the client. I focused on how I could help the other clients rather than focusing on getting the help I needed.

Around 2003 or 2004, I did get my one year medallion for un- interrupted recovery in GA. Sometime after that, though, I was at an AA retreat in the vicinity of the casino I used to frequent. Alone in the car on the drive home from the retreat,

I had to pass by the exit for the casino. I wanted to go and called my good old sister, who asked, "Oh? Do you have any built-in safeties? You didn't bring your ATM or your credit card?" I said, "No," and drove to the casino.

Originally, I went to one GA meeting a week. When that particular meeting closed a few years ago, I didn't bother picking up another meeting. There aren't many GA meetings around where I live but that never would have stopped me from recovering in AA because after inpatient treatment I went for aftercare quite a distance from home for two years. In fact, the travel didn't bother me because I knew it was what I needed to do to stay sober.

For some reason, GA just seemed different to me. I have had my periods of clean time but didn't talk much about that in the meetings. While I still have a sponsor today, we haven't really talked specifically about my GA recovery in awhile.

About six months ago when my sponsor asked if I would speak at their group anniversary, I told her I wanted to think about it. She didn't know I was gambling and I didn't want to tell her. Here I had been speaking with her almost every day, but had never spoken with her about the intermittent gambling.

After thinking about it, I called her back and wormed my way out of speaking at the anniversary by saying that although I was honored to have been asked, I needed to decline because my GA recovery isn't as strong as my AA recovery. She just said, "OK," and that was it.

Presently, I have less than six months of recovery in GA. Intellectually, I rationalize that I only gamble with friends now and never go alone. While I can say I don't gamble like I used to, that really would be like any alcoholic saying that they only drink beer now. I can try to say that I don't have an obsession or compulsion with gambling but I know that just isn't true. If I was counseling someone like me who told me something like that, I would recognize that their statement was irrational.

So, with twenty-one years of sobriety in AA, my master's degree in substance abuse counseling and my certifications as an employee assistance case manager, a community health nurse and a nurse case manager, I do have a gambling problem I can't control. Now sixty-three years old, even with thirteen letters after my name, I have yet to arrive at that point of desperation with my gambling that I reached with my drinking. It was the fear of losing my nursing license that came along with that desperation which drove me to treatment. That is what finally convinced me that I was through doing it my way and that only happened when I accepted that my way didn't work.

Accepting Where I Am In Life

Coming from an Italian family, I was pretty much introduced to alcohol at a very young age. Growing up, I remember having wine at the kitchen table with my parents and grandparents. It was probably around the age of eleven or twelve that I started drinking. Right away, I knew I was unlike other people because I more or less drank to become inebriated.

Very quickly, within about two or three years, I was drinking three or four times a week in high school. Right from the get-go, I knew I was not like a normal person. Although I knew something was wrong right away, I just thought I would be able to grow out of it.

Originally, I went to college for architecture. I only lasted there about six months, though, because, from day one, I found it very easy to get alcohol there. With a bar right next to the school I attended, I pretty quickly drank myself right out of college.

About a year after leaving college, I was drinking every day. I did that for about four or five years while living at home in my parents' basement. My parents enabled me to drink. They both worked and were never home. My grandparents also lived with us at the time and I was pretty much able to periodically go out, come back and drink.

By the time I was nineteen or twenty, I had already started to hit hospitals for detox on a regular basis. I can still remember the smell of being in detox, year after year, two or three times a year. Back then, it almost felt normal to me to end up there. In fact, there were times that I drank an hour after coming home.

I remember being introduced to Alcoholics Anonymous but only went to meetings periodically. My parents also sent me to an outpatient program which I went to for about six months. Still, I was never able to stay sober for more than a month or two at a time.

Although attending AA sporadically, I was really never a part of AA. I began experimenting with some drugs, cocaine in particular, and around the age of twenty-one, cocaine became a very strong part of my life. Back then, I really thought that if I was not drinking it was OK to use cocaine.

Around this time, I was able to get a job at a beer distributor, which was perfect for me. Alcohol and drugs were always around and I was able to drink on a daily basis for free. I lasted at this job for about two years, but eventually drank myself out of that job, too. Throughout this whole time, I was still in and out of detox, trying to get myself straightened out.

My parents eventually got me a job at a government agency which I was able to hold down for a few months. Still drinking, I was not able to hold it together for long though. While I wasn't actually asked to leave that job because of my drinking behavior, there was a change in political leadership at the time which led to the end of that job.

Throughout this whole time, I had multiple relationships. I drank during all of them and lost two or three girlfriends directly due to my drinking.

Eventually, I met a girl who was a friend of the family. I was able to pull it together for a little while and actually thought I had hit the lottery. I thought that I was going to be able to buy back all those previous years with one big decision: to stay with this one girl.

At about the time I started dating this girl, I got a construction job where I went to work every day. I managed to stay sober for about two years while dating her by working and staying busy all the time. Although I'd periodically go to AA, I was just staying busy with no real connection in AA to keep me sober. While I remember at some points having commitments in AA, I was never, ever really into the program. Basically, I was just doing it to get everybody off my back and to keep this girl.

Although my girlfriend really didn't know the full extent of my drinking, I did tell her what was going on with me and what had happened to me in the past. Over time, the relationship got serious and we eventually got married.

About a year before we married, I decided I couldn't take the construction job I was doing anymore and I decided to go back to school. So I started working at a health club as manager of the gym part-time while going to college. After a few of my friends told me that nursing was a good profession, I began going to nursing school full-time.

For about four years after we got married, we lived with my parents. Later on we bought a house and had a daughter together. Again, I just stayed busy, thinking that I had everything together at this point. I wasn't worried about anybody else but myself really. I felt my wife and I were going to be OK because she was financially secure in her job and I was going to be a nurse. I believed inside that everything I'd done prior to this point was really a wash now; that I had gotten everything together and had gotten out of the hole I was in.

Excelling in school and still keeping everything together, I was able to stay sober for about six years. During this time, I got my nursing license and a job in an ICU. So, now I had a beautiful wife, a nice home, a good job as a nurse, a good financial outlook and a newborn baby at home, but I still wasn't happy.

For those six years, I was going to therapy on a weekly basis without AA and I was sober. Throughout this whole time, though, I had to be busy every minute of every day, otherwise I would be uncomfortable. There were times I went to work so anxious that I couldn't walk. I remember going to work so riddled with fear that I called in sick a block away from the hospital due to my severe anxiety.

The therapist I was seeing finally suggested that I should see a psychiatrist. So, on his recommendation, that's what I did. The psychiatrist gave me a multitude of tests, diagnosed me with anxiety disorder and depression, and started me on some Paxil.

After a while, I didn't think that the Paxil was working, so the psychiatrist started me on Xanax. At that point, I really didn't know much about Xanax and I certainly did not know what I was getting myself into when I was prescribed it. Within six months of starting Xanax, I was up to ten milligram a day, all the while working full-time as a nurse in ICU.

I couldn't survive without the Xanax and began manipulating doctors to get more. Meanwhile, I also had a back problem, so I was manipulating prescriptions for Percocet as well. It got to the point where I needed about twenty Percocet and ten to twelve milligrams of Xanax each day, just to get through the day. Routinely, there were five hundred pills in my house at a time.

For the next two years, I was once again periodically in and

281

out of detox for drugs. This happened regularly, about three times a year, all the while with me working full-time in ICU. Eventually, I drank.

I had some stays on psychiatric wards and remember once being admitted to a psych unit after I had a breakdown in front of my house. Still, I was able to keep my job. I was able to disappear for five days at a time by calling out sick for two days since we worked three days a week. Those two days of sick time really bought me five days off in a row which was how I was able to get through all this without having any obvious problems at work.

Needless to say, during this whole time there were opportunities for me to take narcotics from work, and I did. Not so much pills as intravenous medication. Periodically, I would divert the medication from patients who were on medicated IV drips. Sometimes I did this by changing the bags and putting other stuff in it.

I can vividly remember having one particular patient who was on a very high dose Ativan drip. It was very easy to divert that, so I would take the Ativan home and give myself intramuscular injections of sedatives in my thigh to put myself out of, what I thought, was my misery.

This went on for about six months to a year. I thought I was doing OK, at least on the outside, because I still had my job and was able to go through life. At this point, though, my wife had been getting tired of me going in and out of hospitals. There were times I took pills the very next day from work after being away in detox for a while.

At work in ICU towards the end of my shift one day, I had a seizure, probably due to withdrawing from Xanax. I was sent down to CAT scan and actually admitted into my own unit, where I stayed overnight as a patient, which was kind of embarrassing. I'm pretty sure someone must have known what was going on.

Once while orienting a nurse to my unit, I remember I started to slur my words while one of the nurse managers was around. I noticed my speech went to pot but don't know if there was enough evidence of what I was doing to be confronted.

I always tried to keep any inkling of having a problem hidden. There might have been one day when I was asked at work if I was OK but nobody really said anything about any impairment at work. I mean, I looked healthy and would try to do everything I could possibly do to keep up the persona; keep the mask in place to hide the alcohol and drugs I was doing.

At this point, I started to go to AA again to get sober. My friends in AA all told me that I needed to go away to rehab. One friend actually recommended that I go away for three months to a 12 step rehab thousands of miles away which allowed no contact from the outside world. I had just had a baby at that point and was really afraid of losing my job but I made a phone call and got into this rehab that was highly recommended to me.

Going there was probably the best thing that I did in my entire life because it was there that I was taught how to live life. They taught me to understand what an alcoholic and a drug addict is. Up to that point, I never knew what was going on with me. I just thought that I was crazy. I never really knew that there was something wrong with me and that I was unlike other people.

I stayed in the rehab for three months and came out a new

person. Although my wife was very upset about the whole thing and had enough of this back and forth situation with me, I went back to work with no problems. I tried to get the relationship back together but it had really kind of folded by that time.

During the year-and-a-half after I had gotten back from rehab, I was active in AA, going through the steps and making my amends. Then, like many of us, once we start to feel good, we tend not to do what we're supposed to do anymore. Eventually, I drank again.

So I was back in this periodic cycle of being depressed and drinking once every few weeks. Though I tried to keep it together at my job, I struggled at work. When I didn't drink, I would take pills, sometimes from work. Here I was, back to doing what I was doing before.

Separated from my wife, I moved back to my parents' house and fixed up the apartment in their basement. My wife and I divorced when my daughter was six or seven and I continued to be very depressed, very upset and frustrated with the whole thing. I went back to AA and had to start over again. I got myself a home group, a sponsor, a commitment and started back, from scratch, on June 18th, 2006.

Today, I have a whole different attitude towards people who have issues and problems. Like most nurses, I see very sick people all the time in the hospital, so I try to cherish life. I deal with these types of things on a regular basis so I'm very sympathetic to other people's situations, especially regarding drugs and alcohol.

When we had a nurse at work who got caught diverting medication from another floor a while back, I felt so bad for her; yet I honestly don't know if I would be able to turn some-body in. I think I might try to talk with them and tell them what happened to me. I think it important to tell them that, before they hurt somebody, they could talk to somebody and get help. That was something I had to do when I called my EAP and went out on a leave of absence to get treatment.

I am ambivalent about whether or not it would have helped me if I had been caught at work. In a way, I am so grateful I pulled it together and did not get caught at work because I think that might have driven me totally over the edge. I don't know if I would have been able to handle that. Yet, with all I went through due to my alcohol and drug use, I don't feel like I got away with anything.

Today, I'm actually an active member in AA. I have a home group. I have a sponsor. I'm working the steps. I'm feeling somewhat good about myself and I'm able to function in life. I'm able to have relationships, take the good with the bad, go to work and do an honest day's work.

By doing all this, I have found a new relationship with my ex-wife. I have a great relationship with my daughter. I'm able not to be tempted at work by the things that go on there or situations that might invite me to act out like I used to. I'm able to function at my job in a different light, without being selfish and resentful of my situation. I am able to accept where I am in life although that is sometimes a struggle.

I had been taking online classes to get my bachelors in nursing and, after ten years of taking one class at a time, I accomp-lished that. Afterwards, I had applied to a nurse anesthetist program and gotten accepted, which was a great achievement. Ultimately, I found anesthesia wasn't for me after starting the program and although I sometimes regret that, that's just the way it is. I am able to decipher situations like that today and understand that anesthesia nursing might not be the best specialty for me.

Today, I don't have to rely on drugs and alcohol for situations that might bother me. Like anyone else, I get angry sometimes but have a clear understanding that this is just the way it is. I am living a productive life now and even though it might not be totally what I want, it sure is better than what I had. I am not going back and forth to the hospital anymore for detox.

My Drug Of Choice Was Propofol

I grew up in the country as the middle child, with an older sister and a younger brother. My dad was a coal miner and my mother was a homemaker. My childhood seemed normal until I was nine years-old when my mother died of breast cancer at the age of forty-six. I felt lost. My sister was fourteen years-old at the time and had her circle of friends. My four year-old brother lived with my grandmother and my father worked evening hours.

Frequently, I came home to an empty house. I really envied my friends who seemed to have a normal family – mom, dad, brothers, sisters, dinner on the table, and, most of all, someone to come home to or at least cared when they came home.

I was very resentful because I did not have a mother. To compensate for this, I tried to be the smartest, nicest and most accomplished in all areas of my life. I just thought that if I was perfect, I would be loved, and, thus, started my life as being a people-pleaser.

As a young girl, I spent a lot of time watching nurses take care of my mother in the hospital. Whatever the nurses did seemed to make her feel better, so I wanted to grow up to be someone who could help other people. From that point on, there was never any question in my mind; just a very sure decision that I wanted to become a nurse.

While in nursing school, I spent the summers working as a nurse assistant in nursing homes. I just loved it there and I learned basic nursing care without the obligation of detailed charting. The patients taught me many lessons. When I was not yet a nurse, I had this ninety-nine year old patient who had been a barber. When I came at him with the razor, of course, I just about scared him to death, but he talked me all the way through how to shave a person.

Since I enjoyed working with the older population, when I got out of nursing school I thought I would go into geriatric nursing. I graduated from nursing school in 1979, but didn't go right into geriatrics because I thought I should learn some technical skills first. So, I worked on a medical surgical floor and at twenty-one was in charge of forty-five patients, three licensed practical nurses and three nursing assistants. I think back now to how much I didn't know. At the time, I didn't know enough to be afraid.

I enjoyed talking to and taking care of the patients who, in those days, came in two or three days before surgery for a work-up and stayed a week post operatively. I eventually wanted to see what it was like working in the OR and remember a nurse anesthetist who made pre-operative rounds saying he thought I should go to anesthesia school. Looking for something more, I applied to nurse anesthesia school when I was twenty-three years-old. I continued to feel like I needed to do more, be more and be perfect at everything.

Three months prior to graduation from anesthesia school, I got married. I did very well in anesthesia nursing and continued on my journey to do more and be more. After I had my son and daughter, I strived to be the best mother, the best wife, the best nurse and the best everything.

I really worked hard and liked anesthesia, but everything in it was a rat race. There was the turnover time between the cases and the politics; it was just too much. I can remember being particularly frustrated with one surgeon who would schedule eight to ten children for surgery a day. Our routine was pretty much to take the younger cases first and work our way up to the older patients. This surgeon's idea, however, was that the paying patients came first. So, even if the child was six months old and hadn't eaten for four or five hours, the six month-old without insurance had to continue to wait, until the procedure for the ten year-old with insurance was completed. Things like that just really started to frustrate me and I didn't like that part of the job.

Working as an anesthetist for fifteen years, I had the external appearance of having a happy and wonderful life. I was married, had well-behaved children, a nice home and a six figure income. Internally, I was miserable. I was tired, stressed, and worked long hours. I was having a difficult time attempting to be "perfect." I became depressed and did not ask for help because that would mean I had failed.

Never a drinker, I had also never done pills, and never even wanted to. It wasn't like it was planned, or I had any idea where it came from, but, out of the blue, I started thinking, "I can take care of this depression myself."

Although a lot of people have since questioned me about how someone who never did any drugs or anything else before could all of a sudden start shooting up, all I can say is that's what I had; that's what was convenient; and I saw the fast effects of medications on patients.

I had never slept very well from the start of anesthesia school because I would be concerned about the case I was doing the next day. I was always worried that I was going to do something wrong, which is good to a point, but not if it messes up your sleeping habits and your life.

At the hospital where I worked, the CRNAs were required to take twenty-four hour call and we were allowed to sleep if there weren't any cases. Since I could never sleep in that situation, I got in the habit of setting up all the rooms for the next day's surgery. As I look back now, I see I was the perfect enabler to everyone, including myself. I did all the setting up of rooms because I wanted everyone to like me and so things would just go smoother in the morning. I liked the feeling that I was doing well; yet my motive was really to have everyone like me. I wore my ass out trying to be liked.

The first time I took anything was in December of 1998. It was after a night of being on-call with no sleep that I took fentanyl and it felt wonderful. But I didn't want to feel good; what I wanted was not to have to cope with anything. So, after the first couple doses of fentanyl, I started taking propofol, which is not something you can take at work. You have to take it in situations where you can pass out, so I started taking it home with me.

After two weeks of taking propofol, my husband found me passed out in the bathroom with a butterfly needle still connected to the syringe in my vein. After injecting the propofol, the blood had started coming back out of the line, so my husband was scared to death when he found me. He had no idea I had been doing this.

I said I'd never do it again and he told me if I ever did, he would tell my sister who is also a nurse. Although I didn't want anyone to know about my drug use, I did it at home for a few more weeks before my husband found me passed out again and called my sister. It was my sister who helped me get into a treatment center for twelve weeks where I learned about drug addiction.

The inpatient program worked with other professionals, which helped me realize that I wasn't alone. I had no idea what the

12 steps were about and, although I'd heard of Alcoholics Anonymous meetings, I never knew what went on there. I just thought that drunks showed up there and that I certainly didn't fit into that. In treatment with other professionals, though, I started to feel I did have a problem and needed to be there.

Admission to the treatment center was a very humiliating experience. One of the staff members did a full body search while another observed. They stripped me naked, looked in every crack and crevice which was very humiliating, and made me think that, if I ever get out of here, I would never use anything again. I remember there was a guy at the nurses' station who opened my suitcase and pulled out every piece of my clothing, one by one, and went through everything, even my underwear very carefully, which was very demeaning.

I was in the detox section for one day for an evaluation prior to being transferred to "Cottage B" for twelve weeks. This was my introduction to the 12 steps of recovery. I was instructed to bring The Big Book to the AA meeting; so I arrived for my first meeting with my Bible. That's how much I knew about the 12 steps.

While in treatment, my roommate talked constantly about her mother and blamed her addiction on her "terrible" mother. This was an eye-opener for me because I blamed my addiction on not having a mother.

Feeling that I fit in was a slow process. Although I had surrendered my license during my time in treatment, my thought was that I had only done drugs for six weeks, so I couldn't possibly be a drug addict. This thinking allowed me to really minimize everything.

Another thing that helped me minimize the situation was that I was too ashamed to tell the counselors that my drug of choice was propofol. Back then, there were not many people who had abused propofol and I certainly didn't know anyone who had. So, I told everyone that my drug of choice was fentanyl and stuck with that story all through treatment. How could I tell anyone I liked propofol because it made me pass out and allowed me not to have to think or be involved?

When I got out of treatment at the end of twelve weeks, I thought I was doing well. Everything was hush-hush when I got back to work and I was put in preadmission testing, taking the histories for the anesthesia department. This was a good place for me to work because I didn't have to be around drugs.

I had received my monitoring contract from the nursing board, which had taken about three months, and had their approval for return to work in preadmission testing. Although I was not allowed to be in the OR area, when no one was around I would go back to the OR and take propofol. This started the process of using all over again.

The head of the company I worked for found out what I was doing and told me to resign, which I did. I started following my contract from the nursing board to the letter. It took me a year-and-a-half to find a job as a nurse because of the restrictions on my practice. Finally, I found a job doing tele-phonic triage nursing. That was an excellent learning exper-ience and the wonderful friendships I made there will always be with me. Although I was so grateful for the telephonic nur-sing job, I still wanted to go back into anesthesia. I felt that I needed to prove to everyone that I was not "a real addict."

For five years, I went to meetings to get my paper signed, called a number every day, including weekends, holidays and vacations, to see if I had to have a urine drug screen. I went through all the steps to satisfy the Board of Nursing, but I was not in recovery. When I returned to my chosen career, I relapsed immediately. I knew I could take propofol and not be caught on a urine screen because at that time there was no test for propofol and I had never been honest with anyone about it being my drug of choice.

The anesthesia job I had was away from my family and away from my support system, so I had stopped going to meetings. Basically, I had stopped everything I had been doing for five years and became really sick.

It was a miserable situation that went on for about six months. On many weekends, when I should have been going home to my family, I would stay in the motel room and use propofol. It was such a vicious cycle because I would constantly tell myself I was going to stop, but kept on using.

My hemoglobin went down to six and everyone told me how bad I looked. I remember bringing the drugs back to the motel room where I had a room on the second floor. I was barely able to walk up the one flight of steps to my room; yet I still had to keep doing the drugs.

One weekend, in the throes of all this, I went home and, in church, could not even stand up long enough for a song to be sung. I had to sit down in the middle of it. That's the insanity of this disease. Nothing was stopping me and I had to make it into work because I had to get that propofol.

The day I got caught, I had started an IV hep lock the previous evening in order to use propofol all night long. When I went out to work that morning, I thought I better take the hep lock out because, if I didn't, I would use propofol at work. My next thought, though, was that if I did take it out, I would never find another vein that evening.

So, I went to work with the hep lock in, used propofol in the public restroom of the hospital, passed out and woke up to a group of people staring down at me. I thought it was the end of the world. After doing a urine drug screen which was negative for drugs, the OR supervisor dragged me back to my motel room. I was so humiliated and embarrassed. I was just devastated.

This time, I lost my anesthesia career and I lost my nursing license. I was forced to look at why I took drugs. This relapse, and the consequences of it, saved my life.

That is when I finally realized I was an addict. I came back home, knowing there was no way I could get back to long term treatment like before. But I also knew if I kept going to 12 step and Caduceus meetings, that those meetings would be my saving grace. Although I was really embarrassed to admit I had relapsed, I was glad to be going to the meetings. I wanted to go to those meetings.

I remember someone from Caduceus called me, saying all I had to do was start coming back to meetings. He then said, "We will love you until you learn to love yourself." So that's what I did: I started working on me and figured out how I got to be where I was. I went to ninety meetings in ninety days and got a sponsor.

Finally knowing in my heart that I am a drug addict, I have been sober since October 28th, 2004. I've had a probationary nursing license since 2007 and continue to go to 12 step as well as Caduceus meetings weekly. I also see a counselor and an addiction psychiatrist monthly.

The first sponsor I had was a wonderful woman with multiple sclerosis who taught me how to work the steps. She never used her MS as an excuse, even though she was in a wheelchair. I found that especially admirable because I had played the victim a lot and had lots of resentments, like not having a mother. My first sponsor passed away a couple years ago.

My second sponsor passed away last September after having struggled with lung cancer. I am blessed to have known her.

My husband and I have been married twenty-six years. I know I really disappointed him and he cannot forget what happened. Although I can't change his feelings about my disease, I make amends by staying sober.

I feel blessed that my children have done well, despite what I put them through. I found a spiral notebook my daughter had written in, where she wrote about what my addiction was like for her. "My mom has always said how hard it was for her growing up without a mom and she has done the same thing to me because she's not here."

Reading that sentence really hit me hard. Although I never told her I read it, I think she needed to write it and I needed to read it. Knowing I had put the drugs before my family reinforced the power of my addiction and my desire to remain sober.

After being in treatment and seeing the family side of addiction at work, I know that when you go through things as a family, the children are usually stronger because they learn how to cope by using positive skills rather than trying to cover things up. This helped me open up more to my children about my addiction.

I have learned that I am not defined by my job and, by admitting my weaknesses, I have become stronger. Currently, I work in the recovery field and have been involved with the development of a physician health program in my state.

Some other nurses and I have started a nurse support group in our area so that nurses have some place to go, confidentially, where they can get guidance, support and share openly. In this way, we hope to help other nurses who have no idea what to do about their addiction and prevent them from getting sicker. This helps protect the public because the longer the nurse is out there with no place to go and no one to talk to, the more potential there is for harm to patients and the nurse.

Many years ago, I went to the annual nurses' meeting in my state and I sat next to a friend at a presentation given by a nurse in recovery. My friend told me after the presentation that she just could not understand how any nurse could get up before an audience and speak about her addiction so openly.

Eighteen years later, at the annual state nurses' meeting, I spoke about my own experience as an addict. This same friend came up to me afterwards and said, "I understand now that if you can be a drug addict, then anyone can be a drug addict." I definitely get the feeling that God has left me here for a reason.

I Wanted the Whole Package Deal Back

It was my personal life that took the greatest toll due to my alcoholism but I never saw that until the end. I was very successful at work and all my little plans for what I wanted to do in life were getting crossed off my list. My job made me believe I was normal, so I viewed everything that happened to me as if I was a victim.

I was five years-old when my mother died. My sister and I were raised by my grandmother who was a very loving person. My father was young and he got married again when we were still little girls. Although I learned to love my step-mother, she wasn't the chocolate chip cookie maker that I wanted her to be.

Both my father and step-mother drank a lot. They partied a lot and fought a lot. Then, on Sunday morning, everything was back to "normal." I think my father probably had alcoholic tendencies as did a lot of other people in my family.

I was the first in my family to go to college. I went into a four year nursing program and borrowed all the money myself to get through college. My father never asked me how I got the money for nursing school. Looking back, he never asked me how I bought my first car, either. Not that he'd ever think that I stole the money for those things, but it never came up in any conversation.

When I was a junior in nursing school, the Navy came and gave their little speech about enlisting in exchange for the Navy paying my last year of college. I talked my best friend into also joining. My big thing was that I wanted to get away, so I did not have to come home every night and every week-end to the beer drinking and fighting. I thought moving away from that whole situation would change how I would live my life.

I never drank in high school and never smoked. I didn't really even drink until I was twenty-one years old because I was afraid of doing things like that. Doing the right thing was always what I thought I needed to do.

After I got my degree, I went into the Navy as an officer. I married my corpsman which, at that time, was not an easy thing to do in the military because officers were not supposed to fraternize with, let alone marry, enlisted personnel.

We both got out of the service after we were married in 1977. My husband remained in the naval reserve and wanted to finish school, while I went to work for the Veterans Administration. We made friends and did a lot of social events. Even back then, I always wanted the social events to center around what we were drinking. It wasn't ever about the food or the people but about the daiquiris or whatever we were going to drink.

Around 1981, I started to think that I had a problem with alcohol. I was attending graduate school at the time as well as working full-time. I found that I would drink and couldn't remember what I had done the night before. I was working evening shifts in critical care and completing my master's thesis. At the same time, though, I was drinking Tangeray and tonic until noon. I would then go into work to take care of open heart patients. I don't know how I got by doing that because, although I don't think I was ever drunk at work, I certainly must have smelled of alcohol.

As time went on, I knew my husband was concerned because I would drink and would frequently be in a stupor. I don't know whether he ever went to Al Anon, but I know that I could vaguely hear him talking on the phone to people saying he really didn't know what to do with me.

I started to avoid friends because I didn't want to tell them why my phone was off the hook. I took the phone off the hook so nobody would call me because I knew if I spoke to anyone they would probably know I was drinking and that I was drunk.

We were married for five years before we had my son in 1982. I don't remember drinking through that pregnancy but when my daughter was born in 1986, I remember I drank every day throughout that pregnancy. I don't think my husband knew I was doing that, but I was. I prayed to God she would be OK when I went into labor.

In the back of my mind, I somehow knew there was a problem but I couldn't really accept it. I had this attitude that I was still the victim. I just wanted to drink like normal people, go to Happy Hour and be a young adult. So I would go to church on Sunday and pray that God would teach me how to drink; not that He would keep me from drinking, but that He would let me drink like normal people.

One weekend, when my husband was away with his naval reserve unit, I woke up out of a stupor. I had no clue where my four year-old son and one year-old daughter were. I tried to rack my brain as to whether my husband had taken them to a babysitter or whether I had taken them somewhere.

I didn't know what to do but I just continued pretending that everything was OK. I found out later on that the kids had wandered outside on their own and that my son had taken my daughter to a neighbor who was somehow able to get in touch with my husband. Somewhere along the line, Child Protective Services got involved.

My husband and I had some serious issues by this time and I wanted him to move out. I really thought he was my problem and thought I would be able to drink like I wanted to if he moved out.

Around this time, I got involved with a male nurse at work. I thought he was going to solve my problems. Deep down, I really knew I still loved my husband, but the desire to drink was so great that it consumed me. Since this male nurse also drank, he gave me the approval to continue drinking that my husband didn't give me. So my husband finally moved out and I had the two kids, who were really babies at the time.

I was a nurse manager and had success at work, even though I continued to drink. But in April of 1988, when I got my first DUI, the hospital that I worked for found out and required me to get into the monitoring program for impaired professionals in my state. Of course, I didn't realize at the time that once you signed up for that program you couldn't just decide you were going to leave it.

At that point, I went into a long-term, thirty-day treatment program, but even then I never stopped drinking for more than a couple weeks. I had it down to a science exactly how long I needed not to drink before I could give a urine sample that would not be positive for alcohol. While I was mandated to Alcoholics Anonymous by the court, I knew enough about AA that I could turn in the required paperwork. I would describe a made-up story of an alcoholic speaker and forge signatures to document my attendance at meetings.

Meanwhile, my husband had moved back in with me and the

kids after my DUI. A few months later, I moved out to live with the male nurse. I look back now and think, "What kind of mother would leave her children to drink?" But I did leave my children and husband to do just that.

Living with the male nurse turned out to be a horror show because he ended up not only drinking but doing drugs. Our relationship was one of those screaming, throwing, smashing kinds of situations. I had gotten a house by myself and the boyfriend finally moved out. Again, this allowed me to think that I was normal because I was able to cross off my list of accomplishments getting a house by myself and I was still making good money.

In January of 1989, my husband and I got divorced. I really didn't want to get the divorce, but I didn't know what else to do. I was still successful and I earned twice as much money as him, so I thought, "How dare he say anything about my drinking?"

Right after we got divorced, I got my second DUI. I never told anybody about it and don't know how the monitoring program never found out. I was never truthful to those who were monitoring me – never, ever.

Six months after the divorce, my husband wanted to move out-of-state, over a thousand miles away from where we lived. I still remember coming out of the courthouse after the judge awarded him sole custody and permission to move. My husband's van was already packed up and he and the kids left that night.

Now I was left with no children and no husband, still thinking that I was the victim. I was still successful at my job despite the fact that I was in the monitoring program. I saw that

301

program as something else that was aggravating me. How dare they tell me I have to do this or that?

Meanwhile, the hospital I worked for developed its own monitoring program which I felt was mortifying. Whenever they wanted to screen me for alcohol, they would take me to the lab in the hospital where I worked. I had a number instead of a name on the lab work for confidentiality, but people in the lab still knew what was going on because they knew they were drawing my alcohol level.

Most of the people at work really wanted to protect me in every way possible. So I was able to create my very own dysfunctional family as a nurse manager with my employees protecting me. If I smelled of alcohol, they told me to stay in my office. If there was a meeting I was supposed to go to, I didn't go and nobody could ever find me. While I never drank at work, I went into work very hung over. At times, I may have been still drunk from the night before.

In July of 1989, a year to the day after I had gotten the second DUI, I got my third DUI. Neither of those charges went to court until quite awhile later. In fact, I was actually in court on the same exact date in two different counties for those two DUIs. The judge in one county didn't know about the other DUI charge in the other judge's courtroom.

My divorce and custody agreement allowed me to visit my kids once every six weeks for an entire week. To do so, I had to fly up north. The agreement also said that I couldn't drive with my children or be alone with them. I was described as a "chronic alcoholic" and "a danger to my children," which was devastating for me to see on an official document. I still did not want to admit that I had a problem.

Eventually, I asked the monitoring program if I could move to the state my children lived in, but they said they could not monitor me out-of-state. Because I also had a nursing license from the state I was originally licensed in, I was able to work it out so that I reported to that state's monitoring program even though I would be residing in another state.

When I relocated, I had to be involved in outpatient treatment and group therapy and turn in urine screens, all of which was reported to the monitoring program in my initial state of licensure.

To get my transfer within the hospital system in my new state of residence, I had to go back to being a staff nurse. This was a big adjustment for me because by this time I had been in management for six years. Being able to stay in management all those years really allowed me to still think I was a success.

While I started doing a lot of what I was told to do in monitoring, I still wasn't completely truthful. When I was almost finished scamming the monitoring program for the three years I was required to be in it, they found out I hadn't been truthful and my time in monitoring started all over again.

Then when I was not only driving under the influence but driving without a license, I got my fourth DUI. I still thought, "Poor me; how could another bad thing be happening to me?" I still can't tell you what I was thinking but I certainly wasn't overly concerned at the time.

The lawyer told me that I would be released on my own recognizance. I remember I went into work before going to court for this fourth DUI wearing my usual nurse manager attire: a business suit and my lab coat.

When I got to court, the lawyer wasn't there and the judge told me that I had to go to jail. I actually had the nerve to tell the judge, "I can't go to jail. I'm a nurse manager and I have to go back to my job."

Well, that threw the judge right over the edge. He called me "arrogant" and off I went in my heels and business suit and little lab coat to be put in one of those orange outfits, handcuffed to the other women in this dungeon-like place. Then, I was taken off to jail.

The one phone call I did get to make was to my dysfunctional employee family who then fabricated some kind of lie for me. They said that I had a death in the family and had to leave work suddenly, when, in reality, I was sitting in jail.

I didn't know what to do or how to get out of that because I was there without bond or bail set. I spent about a week in jail until my lawyer could get me out. Even after all of this: losing my husband, losing my kids, being in jail, filing for bankruptcy at some point, a psychiatric admission thrown in somewhere along the way, I still thought that I was "OK."

I convinced my ex-husband that I wasn't drinking anymore and wanted to live near the kids. Deep down I loved him and there was still a connection between us. I never told my ex-husband any of my legal troubles and proceeded to move in with him and the kids.

Of course, I kept drinking, which he put up with for about eleven months. During this time, I was sending reports to the other state monitoring program about my AA attendance. I had actually started going to the meetings now, but still hadn't stopped drinking.

Finally, my ex-husband said he couldn't do this anymore and I had to get my own place. So, I got my own place, moved out, and continued to drink. Whenever I would start sobering up, I would take another drink.

Living on my own again, I was doing all sorts of things I never thought I would ever do. I slept with tons of people, not even knowing who half of them were. I worried at one point about HIV because I had no idea half of the time who I was with. I wasn't even able to show up for Christmases after I moved out because I couldn't function without having a drink. I remember I got a tree for my apartment one year, but it stayed in a corner because I never decorated it.

For awhile, I actually carried a shaker of garlic powder in my car. If I thought I smelled like alcohol before I went into work, I would throw a handful of that in my mouth. I do not know whether it was worse to smell like gin and tonic or a bowl of spaghetti, but that was my solution.

I don't know how I ever managed to get through a day because it got to the point where I would break out in a sweat as soon as I got to work and couldn't control my hands to write out report. When I look back now, I don't know why somebody at my job really didn't see what was happening. Maybe they did and just did not act on it.

With only a few dry spells when I was on some kind of diet, I continued going to outpatient treatment and drinking. One week I skipped therapy altogether and the next week I was late for my appointment. I had been out to lunch drinking wine before I went to therapy and the therapist asked for a urine specimen which, of course, was positive for alcohol.

The therapist wrote a letter to the monitoring program which moved the process to the next level. I was put out of the monitoring program and disciplinary actions were brought against my nursing license.

I was supposed to go back to serve a month of jail time in my former state of residence related to the fourth DUI. Instead, it ended up being a two-and-a-half week sentence because I got credit for being in the monitoring program. I drove over a thousand miles to serve my jail term and told the hospital that I was taking vacation to cover the time I spent in jail.

Professional misconduct charges were brought against me by the state that initially licensed me saying that I was not competent to practice. Meanwhile, I had to go for a hearing in front of the Board of Nursing in the state which had first begun monitoring me.

One morning in January of 1994, I had a car accident on the way to the VA which was not alcohol related. I drank that whole week after the accident, taking cabs to liquor stores and sleeping with the cab drivers. That's how my life was, even though it is hard for me to believe now.

During that week, I found out that someone I'd been in therapy with was celebrating a year of sobriety. I just couldn't understand how he got sober because we used to actually go out to drink after therapy. Even so, I went to his first anniversary, probably drunk. That was just a couple weeks before I finally put the drink down.

Then I woke up one morning with vodka bottles everywhere, looked in the mirror, and said, "This is not the person I was meant to be." It wasn't any of the losses in my life that got me to stop drinking. It wasn't the divorce, it wasn't the loss of my children, it wasn't any of that stuff that could stop me from drinking. It was the loss of myself. So I pleaded, "OK, God, if you will help me stop drinking, I'll go to AA. Just help me and I'll do whatever I have to do!"

That very night, there was a snowstorm and I walked to an AA meeting. That was February 7th, 1994, and I made a promise that I would go to at least three meetings a week. I got a home group, a sponsor and a commitment.

Sober just a few months, I went before the nursing board in July of 1994. Although I went by myself, I had an attorney in my state of residence who coordinated things for me. I actually called this lawyer, knowing nothing about him, and came to find that he was sober for twenty-five years at that point after having almost lost his law license. This was a God-send for me and I know that it was Divine intervention.

Having no idea if I was going to come back north with a nursing license after that hearing, I knew that whatever one nursing board decided to do, the other board was going to take the same action against me.

I came out of the hearing with a suspended license with three years of probation. I didn't actually lose my license and could work as a nurse, but I had to get honest with my employer about my license being on probation for the next three years. There was lots of paperwork and reports required of me at that point and I thank God I was sober then. Even so, it wasn't an easy road to get to that point.

Being very quiet in AA my first year in sobriety, I really just sat and listened. After celebrating my first anniversary, I felt like I should do ninety meetings in ninety days because I now had a little bit of a foundation. So, I went around to a lot of other meetings and heard a lot of other people's stories. I also stayed close to the lawyer in recovery who became more like a friend to me. We remained close all these years, up until his death in 2009.

People were put in my life at work and then I'd see them at meetings. I began to have that recovery connection at work. Some people at work knew about my alcoholism because they knew about my three-year license probation. While I'm sure some other people at work knew that I had some kind of trouble with drinking and that I was in recovery, I never made any big announcement or anything about it. I just continued to be involved in AA.

I really believe I could not become sober until I could give up, by getting to that point of acceptance and involvement with AA. It's just like what you read about in the Big Book of Alcoholics Anonymous. My story is in there, over and over again, and that connection I have to the other people in AA is truly a gift and a miracle.

Everything that I had to do for the disciplinary action on my license I did. I made it through those three years with success-ful completion of monitoring. If you look up my license on the computer, of course, it still says that disciplinary action was taken against it. I also got through the probations for all the DUI charges and didn't get into any more legal trouble, although my driver's license is permanently revoked in the state where I received the four DUIs.

Once my professional life was back on track, I looked at my family life. I really wanted to be back in this family, living as a mother with her children. It wasn't like I wanted to go after custody of the kids though, because what I really wanted was to have the whole package deal back: my children and my husband, who I had never stopped loving.

Finally sober, I could understand why my ex-husband had to do what he had done. I had made him out like this terrible person who did this to me, and took my kids away, when all he had done was what he had to do to protect himself and the kids. Of course, I couldn't see that until I got sober.

During my drinking, I had been estranged from my only sister and my family for a while. Somehow, over time, those relationships were also repaired.

When I was sober awhile, I moved into the apartment next-door to my ex-husband for a couple of years. Everybody just laughed about the situation because we always ate together while I lived in the apartment next-door.

After a few years, there was a house on the corner for sale with an apartment in it. I suggested to my ex-husband that we look at it so I could live in the apartment and he could live upstairs. He agreed and we made a bid on that house, but didn't get it.

Since he was willing to consider that, though, I was on a mission to find another house where all of us could move in together. That became part of my focus of recovering my family along with myself. Later on, I found this house that we both liked and we moved in. Somehow living separately didn't last very long.

Although we got back together, I always wanted to remarry my ex-husband. I really wished we'd remarry on what would have been our anniversary date, March 19th. Every year, I would hope maybe we'll get remarried on our anniversary, but my ex-husband never said anything.

In 2002, I was to have major surgery on my back with two

rods inserted for scoliosis. I planned to have that surgery just after what would have been our twenty-fifth wedding anniversary. At this point, I was sober several years, we were living together and everything was truly great.

So on March 18th, 2002, the day before what would have been our twenty-fifth anniversary, I asked my ex-husband, "Are you going to marry me tomorrow or what?" I wasn't really thinking anything would happen, but when he said, "Yes, I'll marry you tomorrow," I told him, "Well, you better mean it because if you say 'Yes' I am going to make it happen."

This was at six o'clock in the morning before he was going to work and I was off for a couple days in preparation for my surgery. So after he didn't take back the words that he'd marry me, I had the divorce papers faxed from the state we were married and divorced in. We met at lunchtime to apply for a marriage license and the next day, March 19th, twenty-five years to the day after we were first married, we got married again with the kids present.

All this was several years ago now and I thank God that my children survived all this. I am grateful that they were taken away before they saw some of the worst of my alcoholism and that they were too little to remember some of it.

My children are young adults now and although we never spoke too much about the past, they know I remain very active in AA and still go to meetings. Actually, it wasn't until I read my daughter's essay to get into college that I even knew she had feelings about my recovery. The essay she wrote was about me and what my recovery has meant to her.

Several years ago, I went to a seminar on addiction in nursing because I wanted to get a nursing license in the state we've lived in for some time. I had such fear of having to relive my past with another Board of Nursing and having somebody think I wasn't OK. I learned about the peer assistance program at the seminar, though, and wrote the nursing board a long letter.

It took a very long time, about nine months, before I ever heard back from them. I had to send documents from the other states I was licensed and monitored in. It was because of that presentation, though, that I thought if I did get a nursing license that I would apply to volunteer for the peer assistance program here. I was hoping that my experience might help other nurses who had drug and alcohol problems.

So, at the age of fifty, I got my nursing license in the state I'm living in and also became a peer assistance volunteer. I felt in that way I could give something back to other nurses with an alcohol or other drug problem. Depending on the nurse I am talking to, I might share a little bit of my story because I don't want them to think I don't know what they're going through. Being a peer assistance volunteer has been very rewarding to me.

I know that my sobriety is a gift. I feel God gave me a lot of opportunities that I just shut the door on because that whole obsession of having to drink was more important than anything else in my life.

It is still unbelievable to me that one day I woke up and just said, "OK, God, if you will help me stop drinking, I'll go to AA. Just help me and I'll do whatever I have to do!" To this day, I never broke that promise I made to God in February of 1994. I'm very grateful I never had to pick up a drink again.

Yellow Rose of Texas Sober Thirty-Five Years

Priscilla was born on November 30th, 1941. Ever since the first time she ran away from home at the age of two, she wanted to move. Priscilla always had wandering feet.

Back when she was growing up, women were really expected to be either secretaries or nurses. Since Priscilla's mother said she should become a nurse, that's what she did. In fact, her sister also went on to become a nurse.

After high school, Priscilla attended a three-year nursing school which was based in a hospital. When she completed the program, she got her first job as a nurse at that same hospital. Although she stayed there for a little awhile, she still had wandering feet and wanted to do something different.

So in 1961, Priscilla decided to enlist in the army. She completed her basic training in Alabama and was then transferred to Fort Sam Houston in Texas, where she began working in the operating room. We met there in November of that year as I was on tour in the army at the time.

I remember when we started dating I asked her if she would like to go out to a movie or something. She said, "You have a car?" The minute I said, "Yes," she said, "Sure, I'll go." After that, when I would go to the field for extended periods to set up tents for officers or take part in make-believe skirmishes for training purposes, Priscilla would keep my car all week long.

One time that I returned to my car is especially memorable. The first thing I noticed was a fan belt sitting on my steering wheel with a note from Priscilla, which said, "Hi. When you get the car fixed, come and pick me up."

Priscilla completed her operating room training in Missouri and was transferred to Colorado after that. When we got married on June 9th of 1962, I was stationed in San Antonio and Priscilla got a transfer back to Fort Sam Houston.

Shortly after that, Priscilla became pregnant. Back in those days, women couldn't stay in the army once they became pregnant, so she was honorably discharged in November of 1962. A month later, she had a miscarriage.

For awhile, Priscilla worked in a doctor's office. Later, she went on to work at other jobs in the nursing field. When we were transferred to the east coast, she returned to work in the operating room as a nurse. In the course of caring for one of those cases, she got stuck by a needle. No one was aware at that time that the patient had hepatitis but when Priscilla developed hepatitis, she didn't work for awhile.

When the first U.S. combat units were deployed to Viet Nam in 1965, I got orders to go to Japan. At that time, Priscilla moved back home to be near her family. She began working at a hospital there until she could join me in Japan.

Arriving in Japan in 1966, Priscilla didn't have a job and, although I didn't know it at the time, she made her job drinking. Alcohol was very inexpensive in the military. Back then, you could get a mixed drink for ten cents, yet a coke in the same size glass would sell for fifteen cents. In those days you could buy a fifth of whiskey for a dollar.

So, while I was working as a medic at the hospital taking care of casualties, Priscilla was spending her time at the house or at the park. We had hired a babysitter for forty dollars a month who washed the clothes and cleaned the house for Priscilla. This gave her more time to drink.

After awhile, Priscilla decided she wanted to go to college. Since she had been in the military, she could get in under the GI Bill, which would pay for her schooling. When she started to go to the university, her initial intent was to get a degree in either social work or psychology.

When we returned to the states in 1968 after spending three years in Japan, I was stationed in Virginia. Priscilla was still drinking but I wasn't aware of it because of the way my job was. She was a closet drinker and I knew nothing at all about alcoholism back then.

In 1970, I received orders to go Viet Nam for a year. While I was there, Priscilla would take our first daughter to the babysitter or preschool. Then she would go to her college class, come home, do her homework and pick our daughter up from school. After that, Priscilla would start drinking and continue for the rest of the day, until she passed out. Her drinking was a problem but I still didn't know about it because I was in Viet Nam.

During my R&R in Hawaii, Priscilla came to meet me. While there, we were staying at my brother-in-law's house. I remember Priscilla drank so much that she got plastered one night and threw up all over the floor. At the time, I thought to myself, "I came all the way from Viet Nam for this? I should have gone someplace else."

So, I talked to her and said, "Priscilla, do you have a drinking problem?" She said, "Oh no. I'm fine." That was it. When my R&R was over, she came back to the states and I went back to Viet Nam to finish my tour.

When I came home in May of 1971, Priscilla said, "I've got to tell you something." She went on to tell me that she was an

314

alcoholic. She told me that she had gotten so bad that one day she wanted to run her own car into an oncoming car, just to kill herself. Instead, she went to church and saw a friend of ours there who talked with her. It was then that Priscilla stopped drinking. She started attending Alcoholics Anonymous meetings and had stopped drinking about a month before I came home.

We've always been partners in things and we continued to stand side-by-side. Priscilla stayed sober and pursued her education. She got an associate's degree and then went on to get a bachelor's degree in social work. She became very interested in working with alcoholics and did her internship in an alcohol treatment program. After she got her bachelor's degree, the program hired her on the spot because they were very impressed with her.

After working there awhile, Priscilla came home one day and said she had this great idea: she wanted to work with the churches. So she became the person in charge of the alcohol counseling service at the Baptist church for the next year-and-a-half to two years.

Priscilla always believed very strongly in maintaining the confidentiality of the people she worked with. We both had great respect for confidentiality because of the military and both of our backgrounds. I remember one night, we went to a Baptist meeting and the preacher was saying he didn't have any alcoholics in his church. Priscilla just tapped me on the shoulder and whispered, "I can't tell you who, but I am taking care of five of the people in his church."

After a time, Priscilla went on to get her master's degree and was hired as an alcohol counselor at the local psychiatric hospital. She no longer seemed interested in clinical nursing positions and quickly rose to being the senior clinician at the hospital. Sometimes she would come home, saying, "It was a rough day, but it was a good day."

Meanwhile, Priscilla kept going to AA and taking it One Day At A Time. She started teaching at the community college, continued to hold groups and became a private practitioner specializing in alcoholism. When she went to work, she could barely get in the door without someone coming to her, saying, "Priscilla, I got this problem." She once told me it got to the point where she was sneaking in the back door at work just to get to her office to be able to put her coat down.

There is a strong history of heart disease in Priscilla's family and on the plane back from visiting family in 1999, she had a heart attack. The plane made an emergency landing and she was brought to the hospital where she had successful open heart surgery. I went up there and we came back home when she had recovered.

Priscilla maintained her sobriety and continued to work with alcoholics. As time progressed, the stress started getting to her and she retired for medical reasons around 2001. We moved up north at the time to where she is originally from until circumstances required me to come back to take care of a brother with cancer.

In February of 2006, we both flew up to New England to visit her family. While we were there, Priscilla felt a lump in her breast. After coming back home, we immediately got in touch with a good friend who was an oncologist.

Although Priscilla always said in all seriousness that she would be hit by a drunk driver driving an eighteen wheeler before she would get cancer, she was diagnosed with inflammatory breast cancer. She was started on chemotherapy but since she got very sick on the medication, they didn't give her all the chemotherapy medication.

When Priscilla developed a high fever in October of 2006, she was admitted to the hospital with a staph infection. During her three week stay, the doctor said he had good news for her: that her cancer was gone. We praised the Lord for that and the doctor said he wanted her to go home and build up her strength.

At her check-up in February of 2007, the doctor told Priscilla that the cancer was back. At the time, she had a radical mastectomy which was followed by a post-op infection. Although the cancer had not really spread, Priscilla decided she no longer wanted chemotherapy. While she was sick, I would take her down to AA meetings and I would attend Al-Anon meetings.

Priscilla had thirty-five years of sobriety when she passed on the 25th of May, 2007, at ten after two in the afternoon. She had stuck by me all those years, even when I was unbearable with PTSD after the war. Even though I had gone from a medic in the army to an LPN, and later became an RN, Priscilla nursed me back to health when I was injured on the job after being kicked in the head by a patient.

Priscilla and I have three children, ten grand-kids and two great grand-kids. Although Priscilla loved her family dearly, she knew it was time to go and that was it. I was right there at her side, along with her sister. The kids came over afterwards and we made all the arrangements for Priscilla to be cremated. Her ashes were taken back to New England where they were buried.

Over the years, Priscilla had met a whole lot of people I never knew about. At the funeral service, the church was completely full of people who I had never met. There were also former staff members she had worked with over the years. Each person at the service came in and told me, "Your wife helped me so much." I never had to ask any of them what she had done for them because I knew fully what Priscilla did for people.

I have bought only three cars in my life. Priscilla bought every other car I ever got. We had a good marriage. I cannot complain at all. She was my Yellow Rose of Texas and I miss her very much.

A Dimension Very Few Ever Achieve

Rachel B. was your Florence Nightingale type of nurse: professional, caring, faithful and loyal. She was also a true lady. Rachel elevated the standard of nursing through her work with fellow nurses, her work with patients and her work at the legislature. She held in confidence all personal matters that were submitted to her keeping. She was devoted to the welfare of those committed to her care. Rachel can never be replaced and we have lost a true professional nurse and a true compassionate person. Rachel was a true friend to all she befriended and to nursing. We miss her deeply and it is our privilege to have known her as a friend and to have her as a friend and colleague.

According to her husband Bill, what really describes Rachel best was what was said by a fellow named Steve whose life had sunk about as low as one can go; a fellow who, at the point when he was just out of prison, was not particularly liked by a lot of people. Somehow Rachel could take the lowest of the low and work with them when no one else would. She sort of took him under her wing and he now has about five years of continuous sobriety.

Steve gave the following oration at Rachel's funeral: I've known Rachel for a little over five years. When I first met her, my life was in ruins. Yet, she invited my wife and I into her home with all the warmth of old friends. Never did I feel one moment of a condescending attitude or judgment for the mistakes I had made in my life; just acceptance and encouragement.

Through the years, we enjoyed many a meal together, the four of us, usually at a local place called The Farm Table. Rachel and I enjoyed greatly the big steaks smothered in the unhealthiest gravy imaginable. Those were good times that will long live in our memory.

She was working gruelingly long hours at the hospital when we first met. I know she was an excellent nurse who cared about her profession. She proved this to us when she was so supportive to our daughter when she was struggling through nursing school. No one could have been so enthusiastic about such a long career unless they really loved what they were doing.

Of course, she had to retire a few years ago when cancer turned her from caregiver to patient; but what a patient she was! I never once heard a word of complaint or discontent about anything they put her through. The chemo, radiation and chemo again; the harsh drugs and countless trips to specialists in Baltimore or elsewhere; no complaints did I hear.

In fact, in those later days I often called to chat with her on the phone, always thinking what I could say to cheer her up. It was a wasted effort and she always answered me with a smile and that funny little laugh she had. I don't think I ever cheered her up one bit; yet she always cheered me up.

Rachel was a special person; the kind you only meet once in a lifetime. Giving beyond her means, caring not just for her friends but people who she had no connection to other than their need for love, support and encouragement, she was fighter for the underdog.

I know from experience that most people bail out of a friendship when hard times come or when life deals a bad hand, but not Rachel. She based her love on a person's heart, not their actions; not their wealth or status in the community. The more unlovable a person was the more she seemed to care about them.

Most people would have given up when they received her diagnosis. The cancer was terminal. Everyone understood that, especially her. She undoubtedly foresaw the pain and suffering that might be in her future, yet she never gave up. Not until the cancer had done its worst to her body and made it impossible to fight any longer. She was a champion of champions. She ran a race far more challenging than any marathon runner ever imagines. One has to ask, how? Where did she find the strength to achieve what she did?

Rachel wasn't an overly religious person but she was an extremely spiritual person. She trusted her Higher Power. It was that Higher Power and her love for Bill and family that gave Rachel her strength and determination to fight.

And fight she did! She stayed with the husband she loved until her body just couldn't take another breath. She couldn't speak in those last moments but I know beyond doubt that her last thoughts were about Bill's welfare and as Bill's friend that was my concern as well.

They were so much in love, still after so many years of struggles together. How could he go on without her? That had to be primary on her mind. I can't explain it but shortly after she passed, I told Bill I had found a peace about it that he would make it. Granted, it would be the most difficult thing he had ever done in his life but he was going to be alright. I believed it then and I believe it now. Maybe that peace of mind was what Rachel was waiting for as well because I know she would never have gone if it meant hurting Bill.

The bible promises that heaven is a place where there will be no mourning, no suffering, no pain anymore; for these former things have passed away. Rachel fought a good fight and she suffered more than we will ever know. As much as I miss her laugh and those meals together, others will miss her even more. Still the pain is ours now. That is always for her. She will suffer no more and for that I am very glad.

We will miss you, Rachel. You were an angel while you were here. Now, you are with the angels holding a place for us sinners, who one day hope to see you in heaven. Thank you for touching our lives. Your friend, Steve.

Briefly describing Rachel's life both leading up to as well as in recovery, her husband, Bill shares:

Drinking brought us together. I think Rachel was probably addicted to me and I was addicted to intimacy with her. Of course, the alcohol fueled all that.

Rachel gave up her career to move to where I was stationed in Key West to marry me. I never felt like I deserved her love but I think addiction played a major role in bringing us together, which happens a lot.

My drinking got so bad in 1990 that I had to go to treatment in detox. While I was in treatment, she came to the family visiting and group sessions. Rachel heard one of the counselors say that I would have to have an alcohol-free home, if I was to survive. At that point, her drinking hadn't gotten nearly as bad as mine.

Rachel was younger than me and had not been drinking as many years but she still abused alcohol. So, she came home and really tried not to drink but couldn't do it. I think she said she lasted two weeks and went back to drinking.

Then, when she came down for the next family group session, she realized that she wouldn't be able to give me an alcohol-free home. So she came forward to the staff and asked them for an evaluation, which I would never have done at that stage. Even that showed a lot of humility on her part and much love for me.

The counselors told her that she really needed to go to outpatient treatment. We were short of money, so she came home. I had two kids in college, one in Harvard, and insurance would not pay for treatment anywhere except at the hospital where she was the Director of Nursing Quality Assurance.

As embarrassing as it was for her, she went to outpatient treatment at our local hospital. Of course, it wasn't very private and I'm sure there was some gossip, but she kept her head high. She never took another drink after her first Alcoholics Anonymous meeting which was at the beginning of January, 1991.

We both grew in recovery. What was once addictive love became really a much deeper love. I grew to love her more and more. All the mischief in our early marriage was gone and the last ten years of our marriage was just wonderful. We went to some meetings together as well as some meetings separately

Rachel grew spiritually more than I did, though. She just seemed to have an innate talent; an insight into taking people under her wing and helping them. The more down and out a person was, the more despicable in society's eyes, the more she seemed to care for them. She looked into their heart and she just didn't give up on people – ever.

Her spirituality grew over her nearly two decades of sobriety. There was just something about her. You just couldn't help but notice when she entered the room. This is not just me talking, though. Other people have told me that an almost physical change would take place in the room when she entered.

Rachel had a profound trust in her Higher Power. She really had a faith that not a lot of people develop in their lifetime. I'm still working on my faith and trust in God and don't know how she developed that.

When she was young, she called herself a secular humanist. Of course, people who call themselves secular humanists tend not to believe in God; yet they believe spirituality can be developed without a Higher Power. But in 1990, something happened to Rachel: she had a deep and effective spiritual experience. She changed; and when she changed, it was like the same old Rachel, yet her heart was different.

I don't want to make her out like she was perfect, though because she definitely was not. She was bow-legged.

Back in the 1970s, I took her to meet my mother and dad. Later, my mother was talking to my sister, Beverly. My mother described Rachel to Beverly, saying, "Rachel is perfectly beautiful, but she's bow-legged."

Well, a few years later when my sister finally told me that story, I went straight to Rachel and told her because at that time in my life I was not very good at keeping a secret. Then, for the next twenty years, I teased her. I'd say, "Rachel, we tried to keep it a secret from you." She would always give me the finger, just flip me the bird, for telling her she was bow-legged. She'd say, "Yeah, and you couldn't wait to come straight and tell me." That became quite a family joke.

Rachel had a wonderful sense of humor. She wouldn't tell a lot of jokes but she liked to hear them. She was a member of the "CIA," otherwise known as Catholic Irish Alcoholic and she was always writing emails to the White House or the state governor, raising hell about something.

She never tolerated hypocrites; was always devoted to her family; strongly advocated for national healthcare; and would get totally disgusted with those Hollywood movie stars who advocated for the rights of pets and animals over the rights of human beings. She always said, "We need to love and take care of our pets but human beings must come first, before animals."

Rachel went to the women's prison and made a lot of 12 step calls. Sometimes she would be worn out in the evening, just absolutely worn out from work, but if somebody called and had a woman in distress who needed some help, she would go and talk to these women, telling them her story. It didn't matter how tired she was. It pissed me off some, too, because I didn't get to see her that night.

I would like to emphasize that something very special happened to Rachel. She had a very deep and effective spiritual awakening that gave her a profound faith in her Higher Power. The faith that she had is of a dimension that very few ever achieve. She never stopped loving me, or I her, truly, deeply, beyond words.

A MESSAGE FROM THE AUTHOR

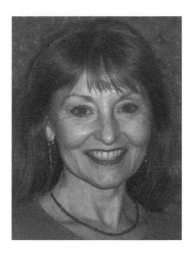

Whether inserting an IV line, presenting on the subject of addiction in nursing, auditing PIXYS usage, making mohair teddy bears or writing a book, I learn best by doing. Over the years, I have come to the conclusion that regardless of what I was taught as a child, practice does not make perfect. Nevertheless, persistent practice performed on a consistent basis can lead one to excel, in spite of challenges.

I have come to accept that the most efficient, economical and relatively painless way for me to realize any goal is to learn from those more experienced; take no shortcuts; exercise self-discipline as well as due diligence; and keep impeccable notes regarding my progress.

These candid accounts clearly demonstrate that permanent, uninterrupted recovery from addiction is possible, even for those who may have come close to death from their affliction in the past. While relapse is a part of some nurses' stories, it is by no means a prerequisite one must encounter in order to recover.

Therefore, it is my firmest conviction that addiction should not be profiled as a "relapsing condition," but more accurately described as a chronic brain disease which is prone to relapse whenever there is disruption or cessation of the actions and attitudes which brought about its remission.

Much help is available for those seeking recovery or in need of support. Some resources which may prove invaluable to some can be found at www.unbecominganurse.org.

Time is our most precious resource. As it waits for no one and there is much work to be done, I will continue to write and present publicly on this critical issue. My primary goal remains the identification and promotion of initiatives which can prevent addiction and relapse, as well as cutting edge strategies which advance nurse safety and wellness.

In the spirit of love and service which Rachel, Priscilla and the other twenty-seven nurses extended to us, it remains my privilege to collaborate with those of you who take a personal or professional interest in this matter. I extend the warmest possible welcome to any who wish to dialogue with me via email at paula@unbecominganurse.org and look forward to networking and brain-storming with many of you in the future.

Warmest regards, *Paula*

ABOUT THE AUTHOR

Paula Davies Scimeca, RN, MS, obtained her baccalaureate degree in nursing from Adelphi University and her graduate degree in psychiatric/mental health nursing from SUNY Stony Brook. Her career has spanned over three decades, with the first ten years spent in medical, surgical and critical care nursing. With over twenty years of experience in addiction and psychiatric nursing, her professional endeavors have been solely devoted to addictive disorders in nurses since 2003. A frequent presenter on the subject of addiction in the nursing profession, she provides strategic consultation services to healthcare facilities and other stake-holders aimed at the prevention and earliest identification of addiction and relapse.

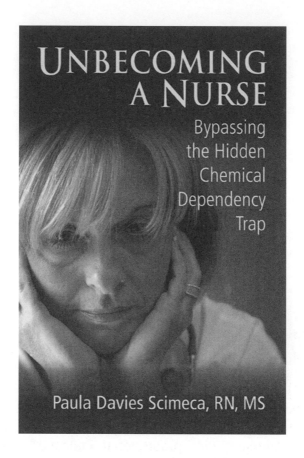

To order copies of "Unbecoming A Nurse: Bypassing The Hidden Chemical Dependency Trap" or "From Unbecoming A Nurse to Overcoming Addiction: Candid Self-Portraits Of Nurses In Recovery" please visit www.unbecominganurse.org or write: Sea Meca, Inc.

PO Box 090455
Staten Island, NY 10309